W9-ARZ-548

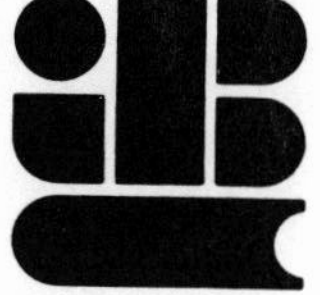

The Future of Allied Health Education

New Alliances for the 1980s

National Commission on Allied Health Education

The Future of Allied Health Education

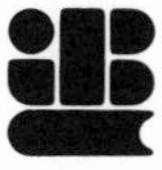

Jossey-Bass Publishers
San Francisco • Washington • London • 1981

THE FUTURE OF ALLIED HEALTH EDUCATION
New Alliances for the 1980s
by the National Commission on Allied Health Education

Jossey-Bass Inc., Publishers
433 California Street
San Francisco, California 94104
&
Jossey-Bass Limited
28 Banner Street
London EC1Y 8QE

Library of Congress Cataloging in Publication Data.

National Commission on Allied Health Education.
The future of allied health education.

Bibliography: p. 259
Includes index.
1. Paramedical education—United States.
2. Allied health personnel—United States.
I. Title. [DNLM: 1. Allied health personnel—Education. 2. Allied health personnel—Trends.
W18 N27715f]
R847.5.N37 1980 610.73'07'1173 79-9666
ISBN 0-87589-457-7

Manufactured in the United States of America

JACKET DESIGN BY WILLI BAUM

FIRST EDITION
First printing: April 1980
Second printing: November 1981

The Jossey-Bass
Series in Higher Education

Introduction

The National Commission on Allied Health Education was created in September 1977 to conduct a two-year study of allied health education in the United States. It was charged with making recommendations for the next decade based on assessment of the developments in allied health education during the past decade, current problems confronting educational institutions that prepare allied health personnel, and current and future arenas for health service. The reference to past and future decades in the charge is appropriate, for the study's inception marked both the end of ten years of remarkable growth and change in a major and vital segment of the workforce and the beginning of a new era for allied health education.

In the words of Robert E. Kinsinger, vice-president of the W. K. Kellogg Foundation:

> This volume is the result of a reassessment and rethinking of the allied health movement in the seventies and a careful consideration of how it might best function in the decade of the eighties to provide optimum health service to individuals. It analyzes past and current issues and responses and suggests policy principles. It further makes concrete recommendations for action programs with specific identification of the agencies and institutions that should take the lead in these actions. It provides the data that were gathered and utilized to arrive at the recommendations.
>
> It should also be noted that the W. K. Kellogg Foundation studied the allied health movement during the decade of the seventies. In some instances, the Foundation provided financial assistance for key developments in the field. This was deemed an appropriate role for a foundation dedicated to the application of knowledge to the problems of people and specifically concerned with new initiatives for providing health care. Changing social, political, and economic forces are beginning to shape a new era for the field of allied health. Thus support for an independent National Commission on Allied Health Education was judged timely.

The commission was totally supported by a grant from the W. K. Kellogg Foundation to the American Society of Allied Health Professions (ASAHP). The proposal specified that: "The commission will be independent of ASAHP in carrying out its study and formulating its recommendations. The commission will be housed in the ASAHP National Office and its relationship with ASAHP will be only for selected administrative services. ASAHP also will serve as fiscal agent for the commission." This "arms-length" but cooperative relationship was maintained throughout this study.

Who's Who of the Study

Ralph H. Boatman, who served as president of ASAHP in 1977, and Frank G. Dickey, chairman of the commission, had the task of selecting fourteen commissioners from a list of over two hundred names nominated from the field in response to a request by ASAHP. At the outset, it was decided that this would be a working commission rather than one designed to do no more than rubber-stamp recommendations prepared for its review. Moreover, it was clear that no body of fifteen members could entirely represent all the groups concerned with allied health education: professional associations, educational institutions, employers, regulatory agencies, practitioners, faculty, students, and the public at large. Consequently, the major criteria for selection were the expertise of the individual and his or her ability to make a substantial contribution to a working commission and to place the broad interests of allied health education above the special interests of particular groups. Obviously, no one is without biases, and wide differences in opinion on many issues, reflecting diverse backgrounds and experiences, led to some lively discussions at commission meetings. The commissioners, and the sectors from which they were drawn, are as follows:

Community and Junior Colleges	Roger Smith
Four-Year Colleges and Universities	Einar Olsen
Medical Schools	William H. Knisely
Trade and Technical Schools	Jack F. Tolbert
Hospitals	Haynes Rice
Medicine	Jack H. Hall
Nursing	Dorothy McMullan
Allied Health Education	Darrel J. Mase
	Nancy T. Watts
Dental Auxiliary Education	Mary Jane Kolar
Laboratory Education	Doris L. Ross
Physician Assistants Education	Donald W. Fisher
Consumer Interests	Ernest Ratliff
Public Health-Community Health	Jack B. Hatlen
Postsecondary Education	Frank G. Dickey

At the second meeting of the commission, Dorothy McMullan was elected vice-chairman of the commission.

In September 1977, the staff began work under the direction of Engin I. Holmstrom, a sociologist who had previously served as policy associate with the American Council on Education. For the position of associate study director, Holmstrom appointed Ann S. Bisconti, a social scientist who had been employed as research coordinator for the University Research Corporation and as an adjunct research associate for the Higher Education Research Institute. Although Holmstrom and Bisconti had some research experience with allied health education, they were purposely recruited from "outside the field." It was hoped that, as outsiders, they would view problems from a fresh perspective, maintaining skepticism regarding certain long-held but unproven beliefs that constitute the folklore of the field. The core staff also included Ida E. Green, who served as administrative assistant. Other personnel were utilized to work on specific projects or as temporary assistants; thus the staff ranged from three to thirteen, depending on the workload.

One of the charges to the commission was to make recommendations based on an assessment of the current and future arenas in which allied health personnel must function. It seemed logical that a future-oriented commission should place its recommendations for education within the context of future health service needs. To provide this context, in the fall of 1978, the commission appointed an Advisory Panel on Health Service Needs. Panel members were asked to do some creative thinking in response to a series of "what if" questions centering on the future utilization of allied health manpower. For instance, the group was asked: What impact would different versions of the National Health Insurance plan have on allied health manpower? What would happen if Health Maintenance Organizations (HMOs) were to serve as many as one fourth of the eligible population? What effect would the so-called physician oversupply have on the utilization of allied health personnel? The members of the Advisory Panel on Health Service Needs were:

Howard L. Bost, assistant vice-president, Albert B. Chandler Medical Center, University of Kentucky

Harriet M. Kriesberg, principal associate, Robert R. Nathan Associates

Marvin M. Kristein, chief, Division of Health Economics, American Health Foundation

John Alexander McMahon, president, American Hospital Association

Richard M. Scheffler, then director, Division of Health Manpower and Resource Development—Institute of Medicine, National Academy of Sciences (now with the Department of Economics, George Washington University)

Stages of Commission Work

In September 1977, the commission staff conducted an informal survey to learn the opinions of a wide range of individuals relating to the major problems facing allied health education today and the major issues for the near future. Included in this grass-roots survey were administrators of allied health programs in collegiate settings, representatives of professional associations, state planners, and researchers. The concerns of the respondents were found to cluster in six major areas: definition and identity, credentialing, funding, roles of educational settings, clinical education, and articulation. Less imperative, but also mentioned, were concerns about continuing education, leadership development (especially for faculty and administrators), student selection and retention, and research and information needs. Some respondents also emphasized that education must be related to the needs of consumers and that improved delivery systems must be developed to meet these needs. One notable finding of this survey was that even though consensus on problems was high, there was no general agreement on solutions. Thus the field looked to the commission for solutions and guidelines to meet the challenges of today and tomorrow.

The work of the commission was conducted in three stages: planning, documentation, and recommendation development.

Planning Stage. Between September 1977 and February 1978, the major effort went into defining the scope of the commission study and specifying the topics to be covered. Of great help in this regard were the results of the grass-roots survey, which—combined with an extensive literature search and review of data sources by the staff—yielded a long list of possible study topics. After three meetings, the commissioners decided on the specific study topics, using the following criteria as guides: (1) that topics be focused on education, (2) that they be amenable to sound documentation, (3) that they relate to areas where the commission could make an impact, and (4) that they not lead to duplication of the work of other groups. For instance, with respect to this last point, the accreditation and credentialing processes were rejected as topic areas because they had been or were being studied by other groups. The focus of the commission was education and not manpower. Manpower requirements and utilization trends would be studied only to provide a broad context for future educational needs, whereas supply and demand for particular occupations would not be assessed. Finally, the scope of what could be done was so large that some priorities had to be set. Although the commissioners felt that there were other issues just as important as those included in the commission study, time constraints did not allow a thorough examination of such areas as continuing education or student selection and retention.

At the March 1978 meeting, the commissioners set priorities on topics for study, which were found to cluster in three major areas:

- *Field-related questions:* clarification of roles and functions of allied health occupations; their identity problems; manpower issues, including services, utilization patterns, and future service needs; organizational and individual leadership development in allied health.
- *Educational settings-related questions:* roles of various settings that prepare allied health manpower; educational program establishment and review in colleges and universities; appropriate educational content; articulation between educational programs and levels.
- *Educational coordination questions:* issues dealing with sharing of resources through interinstitutional collaboration (for example, consortia, clinical affiliations) and intrainstitutional collaboration (for example, interdisciplinary education, core curricula).

In addition to topic selection, certain other basic decisions had to be made. The name National Commission on Allied Health Education itself presented some problems. Which of the numerous health occupations were to be considered under the rubric *allied health*? Which of the many levels and settings for the education of health personnel were to be studied? Should the study examine and address recommendations to programs at all levels, in all types of settings, and for all types of health personnel?

After considerable debate, the commissioners were unable to reach consensus on the occupations to be included under the term *allied health.* Instead, they decided to postpone defining allied health until the documentation studies had been completed. Further, the study was not intended to address specific occupations but rather to identify broad similarities and differences among the occupations and to examine educational approaches and processes of general concern.

Greater clarity was achieved at the start in determining the educational settings to be studied. It was decided to include all formal postsecondary education programs (not only those offered in colleges and universities but also those offered in proprietary schools, hospitals, the military, and other settings) but to exclude high school programs and on-the-job training programs.

Documentation Stage. Between March 1978 and March 1979, staff activities were aimed at providing the commissioners with solid documentation in those areas identified as having high priority for further study. Published and unpublished materials were gathered and analyzed and existing survey data were used to study issues reported in documentation papers, constituting the agenda for four commission meetings. Also during this stage, the Advisory Panel on Health Service Needs met to assess trends in health care and to formulate scenarios designed to serve as a context within which the commission's recommendations on education could be made.

Maximum use was made of existing sources of data on allied health education, particularly the ASAHP and American Hospital Association inventories of educational programs in collegiate and hospital settings. Also useful was the U.S. Office of

Education's Postsecondary Career School Survey. In addition, two formal surveys were conducted: one of the professional associations representing allied health personnel and the other of practitioners and educators in leadership positions (see Appendix A for details). Besides these formal surveys, a number of informal surveys were carried out, using a panel of administrators connected with allied health programs in academic health centers.

Recommendation Development Stage. The recommendations in Chapter Six represent the consensus of the commission. They were developed and refined over a period of five months. Much of the work was accomplished in task force sessions, with each of the three task forces directing its attention primarily, but not exclusively, to those topics that it had initially proposed for study.

Task Force One, under the leadership of Donald W. Fisher, dealt with the general question "What is allied health?" and developed the classification scheme used in Chapter Two to describe allied health services. It was also responsible for drafting recommendations on ways to relate allied health education to practice needs, selection and guidance of students, and continuing education. Task Force Two, led by Jack H. Hall, focused on issues affecting educational settings: determination of appropriate preparation (that is, justification of the level and length of basic occupational preparation programs and control of unnecessary proliferation of these programs), criteria for program establishment and review, articulation, and inclusion of appropriate subject matters in the curriculum. Task Force Three, with Dorothy McMullan as leader, was concerned with collaborative arrangements in education, the integration of clinical and didactic education, and leadership development.

Definitions Used in the Study

The decision not to define allied health at the beginning of the study resulted in three different usages. First, for the purpose of staff studies describing educational programs, all occupations listed in the ASAHP *Glossary of Health Occupation*

Titles were treated as allied health. The *Glossary* lists virtually all health occupation titles that have programs in the collegiate sector but excludes physicians, osteopaths, dentists, veterinarians, optometrists, podiatrists, pharmacists, clinical psychologists, and registered and licensed practical nurses. It includes some nursing categories such as nurse practitioner, nurse aide, and nurse anesthetist (see Appendix B). The *Glossary* was compiled with the advice and counsel of several government agencies and has been used by ASAHP in its surveys of health occupations educational programs in two-year and four-year colleges and universities. These surveys were the major source of information for commission studies of educational programs on which Chapter Four is based.

Second, after looking at initial findings, the commissioners decided to drop from manpower discussions nursing-related categories in the *Glossary* as well as special education teachers. It did not appear reasonable to include some nursing services in the allied health category (for example, nurse practitioner) and to exclude others (for example, licensed practical nurse). Furthermore, to call nurse aides, whose numbers total over a million, "allied health personnel" would give a distorted picture of the types of services performed. Finally, it was felt that all nursing-related personnel listed in the *Glossary* identify strongly with nursing and take their direction from nursing. Similarly, special education teachers (for example, teachers of the deaf, teachers of the emotionally disturbed) should be categorized as teachers rather than health care providers, since their functions relate more to teaching than to health. Chapters Two and Three, which describe allied health occupations and careers, use this more limited definition of allied health.

These two were the operational definitions of allied health: the first for the purpose of educational studies, and the second for the purpose of manpower studies. The third and final definition of allied health was reached after the staff studies had been completed. This definition reflects the commissioners' conviction that all health personnel working toward the common goal of providing the best possible services in patient care and health promotion should be included in the allied health category (see Chapter One). The final definition is a goal to be achieved, however, and should not be confused with the study population, which varies and is determined entirely by practical considerations.

Throughout the study, the term *occupation* is used, as defined by the U.S. Department of Labor, to mean "the name or title of a job which identifies and specifies the various activities and functions to be performed." No attempt has been made to distinguish between professional and nonprofessional occupations. Thus, "physician" and "speech pathologist" are referred to as occupations, as are positions at the aide level.

Similarly, throughout the study, the term *educational institution* is used to refer to both collegiate and noncollegiate settings. Finally, the commission refers to persons prepared in more than one occupational role (for example, as both radiologic technician and medical laboratory technician) as having "cross-occupational competencies" rather than "multiple competencies," since it is assumed that all allied health personnel have multiple competencies.

What Can the Commission Do?

This report has been awaited, we sense, with both hope and anxiety. Not surprisingly, the purposes of this study have been compared by some persons with those of past major studies of various health occupations, most notably the Flexner Report of 1910, which resulted in radical changes in medical education. The current status of allied health education is very different, however, from the state of medical education in 1910.

Complementing a movement toward preparation in the basic sciences, the Flexner Report sought to bring medical education out of the preceptorial tradition and into the university. Today, the preceptorial tradition is a thing of the past for virtually all health occupations that require a solid grounding in science. What has been somewhat neglected and what is needed now for the education of all health personnel is an equal emphasis on the humanistic approach to practice and on concern for the whole patient.

The Flexner Report also sought to upgrade the quality of medical education by consolidating and eliminating programs, particularly commercial programs with poor clinical facilities, and by lengthening preparation. There is no denying that some allied health programs today are of poor quality, but the controls are different. Quality assurance mechanisms exist, and the accreditation process—which is currently undergoing considerable scrutiny by various groups—serves a useful function, particularly in higher education. Coordination is indeed an important goal—above all, to check the unnecessary proliferation of programs—but statewide and regional mechanisms for scrutinizing educational and health-related activities are already in place, and there is good reason to believe that educational institutions will be increasingly required to demonstrate the need for establishing new programs and for continuing existing ones. Given the trend toward regulation of both the health and education systems, any recommendation by this commission for greater collaboration and coordination seems superfluous. What the commission can do is offer guidance on how to collaborate and coordinate, how to anticipate problem areas, and how to identify the factors to consider in program development. In doing so, the intention of the commission is to be enabling rather than regulatory. Moreover, the commission hopes to provide an incentive for self-scrutiny and control, which is the most effective way of staving off the encroachment of governmental regulations.

Chapter One of this volume describes the developments that led to the recognition by the federal government of allied health occupations as a group and discusses the changing concerns of the field. This chapter also presents the problems associated with the inclusion and exclusion of certain occupations within the general allied health category, followed by a brief discussion of the deliberations of the commissioners and their decision regarding what constitutes allied health for the purposes of this study.

Chapter Two presents a discussion of characteristics of

allied health occupations (as defined for the purposes of this study). Clearly, the great variety of services provided by allied health personnel needs to be recognized and stressed. Some services require lengthy and rigorous preparation; others do not. Requiring longer formal preparation than is needed amounts to a disservice to both students and society, and in Chapter Six the commission suggests ways to bring this trend to a more realistic perspective, relating education more directly to practice needs.

Chapter Three discusses the outlook for allied health careers, examining the current trends in manpower patterns as well as socioeconomic and political forces that are bound to have an effect on the preparation and utilization of allied health personnel in the coming decades. The increasingly important role of allied health personnel in meeting the nation's future health goals and priorities is described.

Chapter Four provides a descriptive account of the current educational scene, with information on formal allied health programs in colleges and universities, hospitals, noncollegiate postsecondary institutions, and the armed forces. No information is available on informal on-the-job training programs, on in-service education provided by many health care providers, or on formal programs offered by health care providers other than hospitals. Although the settings for allied health educational programs are numerous and, in some cases, overlapping, each seems to have a unique role in meeting specific service or student needs. Thus the commission does not endorse one type of educational setting over another but recognizes that a wide range of educational modes, corresponding to the wide range of competency levels required for health care, is desirable. Moreover, any reference to "educational institutions" applies to all settings with formal postsecondary programs for allied health occupations.

Chapter Five describes different forms of collaborative and cooperative activities among and within educational institutions. Because of lack of data on other settings, this discussion is limited almost exclusively to activities in collegiate settings. The need for greater cooperation among various types of educational institutions and among educational institutions, professional associations, and health care providers is acknowledged.

Finally, Chapter Six presents the commission recommendations and the rationale for the development of each one. Fifteen primary recommendations are offered as major policy guidelines for future developments in allied health education. These are followed by sixty-three corollaries that provide the means for achieving the goals implicit in the primary recommendations. Not all the recommendations in Chapter Six represent new ideas, nor are all of them action oriented. Some of the recommendations have been heard before but are not universally followed. They are reemphasized here because the commission believes that greater adherence to these policies will improve the quality and efficiency of education and health care. Some of the action-oriented projects or innovative approaches proposed by the commission have been tried before in allied health or in other fields. They are presented in the belief that they should be tried again, implemented on a wider scale, or introduced to allied health education because they have the potential for meeting future needs effectively. It is recognized here that the goals implicit in the primary recommendations of the commission may be achieved through other methods just as effectively; the commission strongly encourages implementation of different approaches.

The recommendations are addressed to a wide audience, including administrators, teachers, students, professional groups, practitioners, providers, federal and state governments, regional planners, and private foundations. Some are of general concern and, the commission believes, should be taken under consideration by many groups involved in allied health education. Others are targeted to particular groups.

It should be obvious from the recommendations that the commission believes that allied health personnel, in their many and varied roles, are one of the nation's most valuable resources. It is essential that their education be effective, efficient, and appreciated. It is hoped that this report will eradicate some unfounded myths and point the way to new directions to meet the challenges of the 1980s and beyond.

The commission has no regulatory or enforcement powers. It can neither wield the stick nor offer the carrot. It is to be hoped, of course, that some of these recommendations will be implemented. But the true measure of the success of the commission lies elsewhere. If the recommendations in this report motivate allied health practitioners and educators to a new self-assessment, if they provoke discussion and debate, if they stimulate efforts, and if they lead to better communication and collaboration among different groups and sectors, then the commission will have achieved a worthwhile goal.

In many sectors of our educational and professional programs, allied health education has not always been accorded the respect that it is due. It is hoped that this study will produce a greater desire on the part of all concerned to bring allied health into the mainstream of postsecondary education. Coordination and collaboration with other more traditional departments within our institutions could bring about a change in the "stepchild" syndrome.

In conclusion, it is important to point out the significance of this report for administrative officers of postsecondary institutions. The commission strongly believes that the time is at hand for a complete reassessment of the allied health programs in these institutions. Funding for such programs is increasingly difficult to obtain and, with the changing demands of society, new approaches to allied health education become necessary. The report of the National Commission on Allied Health Education is designed to serve as a guide for all concerned with allied health education in this period of reassessment and readjustment.

Frank G. Dickey
Chairman of the Commission

Acknowledgments

The past two years have been both challenging and rewarding for us. Working with our capable and thoughtful commissioners has been an exhilarating experience. These fifteen individuals from extremely diverse backgrounds became, over the two-year period, a strongly cohesive unit with an unusual degree of mutual respect and understanding—a model for what we hope can be achieved more broadly in allied health education and services. We can honestly say that this commission focused on issues and problem solving rather than on the promotion of personal agendas. These accomplishments can be attributed in large part to the warm, patient, and gentle leadership of chairman Frank G. Dickey. Moreover, he was unflaggingly supportive of staff and helped see us through various crises with humor and sagacity. Our thanks and affection to Chairman Dickey and all the commission members.

During these years, the commission staff was housed in the offices of the American Society of Allied Health Professions. While always careful to maintain an arms-length relationship to protect the independent status of the commission, they made us feel welcome and provided a congenial work environment which we greatly appreciated. Most important, the research staff, under the direction of Richard S. Nunn, contributed to the smooth functioning of the staff studies by responding immediately and unselfishly to all our data-processing needs.

We were fortunate to have exceptionally well-qualified and dedicated staff associates and assistants. The secretarial and conference-planning skills of our administrative assistant, Ida E. Green, are already legendary. We would like to thank her especially for the many long days of work beyond the call of duty, cheerfully performed. Other staff members, although all part-time, worked on special assignments diligently and wholeheartedly, and all made significant contributions to the study. Through her expert editing, Laura Kent added grace and style to earlier versions of this manuscript and to many of the earlier studies prepared by staff for commissioners' review. She also co-authored an article that reported the staff study of "Grassroots Concerns."

Particular acknowledgment should also be made of the contributions of Jeannie T. Waszilycsak, for her study of allied health education in the armed forces, Ann Schuerman, for preparing materials for background studies on health services and settings, and Naomi Glass, for preparing the materials for the background study of federal funding patterns. Our thanks also go to our student assistants Alex Hamza (Massachusetts Institute of Technology), Melanie Kaye and John Newbery (Georgetown University), and Sarah Johnson (Duke University).

We are especially indebted to Robert E. Kinsinger, vice-president, W. K. Kellogg Foundation. His keen interest in and enthusiasm for the field was contagious, keeping us on course and eliciting our best efforts.

Finally, our gratitude goes to all those in the field who have been so generous with their time and energy, contributing to the commission's work in numerous ways. We have made many friends in allied health and will always remember them fondly.

Washington, D.C.
March 1980

Engin Inel Holmstrom

Ann Stouffer Bisconti

Contents

Tables and Figure

Tables

Figure

Commission Members and Staff

Frank G. Dickey, Ed.D., chairman, National Commission on Allied Health Education, and formerly president, University of Kentucky; provost, University of North Carolina at Charlotte; and executive director, National Commission on Accrediting

Donald W. Fisher, Ph.D., executive director, American Academy of Physician Assistants and Association of Physician Assistant Programs

Jack H. Hall, M.D., vice-president for medical education, Methodist Hospital of Indiana

Jack B. Hatlen, M.S., director, Office for Allied Health Programs, University of Washington

William H. Knisely, Ph.D., president, Medical University of South Carolina

Mary Jane Kolar, M.A., director of education, American College of Cardiology, and formerly director, Division of Professional Development, American Dental Hygienists' Association

Darrel J. Mase, Ph.D., professor, University of Florida at Gainesville, and first president of the American Society for Allied Health Professions

Dorothy McMullan, Ed.D., consultant in nurse education, New York City

Einar Olsen, Ed.D., president, University of Maine at Farmington

Ernest Ratliff, LL.B., attorney at law, Raleigh, North Carolina

Haynes Rice, M.B.A., hospital director, Howard University Hospital

Doris L. Ross, Ph.D., associate professor and program director, University of Texas Health Science Center at Houston

Roger Smith, M.A., vice-president for planning and development, Tulsa Junior College

Jack F. Tolbert, M.A., president, The Medix Schools in Baltimore

Nancy T. Watts, Ph.D., director, Office of Educational Services, Planning, and Evaluation, Education Division, Massachusetts General Hospital

Commission Staff

Engin Inel Holmstrom, Ph.D., study director

Ann Stouffer Bisconti, Ph.D., associate study director

Ida E. Green, administrative assistant

The Future of Allied Health Education

New Alliances for the 1980s

I

The Allied Health Concept in the Next Decade: New Meanings and Challenges

Having been initiated and recognized much later than medicine, nursing, and public health, allied health as a concept is not yet understood and appreciated. It has, however, great potential for promoting alliances in education and health service. As currently used, the term *allied health* is generally applied to occupations whose primary function is to provide health services or promote health. Preparation for such occupations ranges from on-the-job training to postgraduate education. Direct patient care is the main activity of some occupations, such as physical and occupational therapist, whereas others, such as medical technologist, have relatively little direct contact with patients. Still other occupations, such as community health educator and environmental health specialist or sanitarian, deliver services that are preventive in nature.

Development of Allied Health Occupations

Since the turn of the century, the total health workforce has been growing and changing, and this trend gathered momentum in the 1960s. In terms of overall numbers, the growth was staggering: from 345,000 in 1900 (Bureau of Health Manpower, 1967, p. 5) to 2 million in 1960 and 4.3 million in 1970 (Bureau of Health Manpower, 1978, p. II-21). Even more dramatic were the changes in the nature and composition of this workforce. As health service improved and expanded, more types of personnel who had competencies in specialized areas and who could work together effectively were required. Before 1900, only a handful of health occupations existed. At least twenty-seven new occupations—including dental hygienist, dietitian, occupational therapist, physical therapist, speech pathologist, radiologic technologist, and medical technologist—were established between the turn of the century and 1940.

Between 1940 and 1965, many other occupations came into being, including medical record personnel, respiratory therapist, physician assistant, and a variety of technicians and assistants whose functions supported the older allied health categories. In 1900, one in three health workers was a physician (Pennell and Hoover, 1970, p. 3). By 1960, physicians accounted for just over one in ten, and by 1970, just one in thirteen (Bureau of Health Manpower, 1978, p. II-21).

Federal Legislation. Despite these increases in personnel, the need for health manpower continued to grow until, by the mid 1960s, the inbalance between supply and demand became a national concern. Moreover, increased attention was directed to the many health occupations which, as a group, were referred to as "allied health professions." The first Act of Congress directed specifically to allied health education, the Allied Health Professions Personnel Training Act, was passed in 1966. Designed "to increase the opportunities for training of medical technologists and personnel in other allied health professions" and "to improve the educational quality of the schools training such allied health professions personnel," this act provided for grants-in-aid to public and private nonprofit training centers for allied health professions: that is, to accredited two-year colleges, four-year colleges, or universities that were affiliated with a teaching hospital and that offered training for at least twenty persons in specific allied health curricula leading to an associate degree or higher. Grants were awarded for basic improvement and special projects, construction, advanced traineeships, and curriculum development for new types of health care providers. Since 1966, the Bureau of Health Manpower has awarded over $200 million to professions and programs that qualified for federal assistance under the Allied Health Professions Personnel Training Act.

First National Study of Allied Health Education. In 1967, soon after the passage of the Allied Health Professions Personnel Training Act, a report on the first comprehensive national study of allied health education, *Education for the Allied Health Professions and Services,* was prepared at the request of the Surgeon General by the Allied Health Professions Education Subcommittee of the National Advisory Council. This report described the status of allied health education and set the quantitative goal of doubling the output of educational programs.

The subcommittee clearly favored the collegiate sector as the appropriate setting for high-quality education: "Education and training are primarily the business of educators in educational institutions. Education for the health professions must include a substantial portion of clinical experience; yet the character and nature of that experience should be under the control of the educational institution primarily responsible for the program, to insure that the clinical exposure provides the requisite educational value" (Bureau of Health Manpower, 1967, p. 22). This basic assumption led to a series of recommendations for developing allied health education in the collegiate sector. In particular, the subcommittee recommended that coordinated allied health education units be established in colleges and universities, on the grounds that such units promote interdisciplinary communication and cooperation. At the time, there were just ten schools of allied health, nine of them associated with medical centers. At latest count, at least sixty-six colleges and universities have schools or divisions of allied health.

New Organizations in the Mid Sixties. A related development during the mid 1960s was the establishment of two organizational entities that gave further recognition and impetus to the formal preparation of allied health personnel. In 1966, the American Medical Association (AMA) established a Department of Allied Medical Professions and Services, out of which grew the current Committee on Allied Health Education and Accreditation (CAHEA). The AMA had been involved in the accreditation of formal educational programs for allied health occupations since 1933 when, at the request of the American Occupational Therapy Association, it helped to formulate standards for the accreditation of occupational therapy programs. Between 1933 and 1966, it had worked out similar cooperative arrangements to accredit programs for medical technologists, physical therapists, medical record administrators and technicians, radiologic technologists, cytotechnologists, and respiratory therapists. The reorganization in 1966 establishing CAHEA resulted from the recommendations of an AMA Commission to Coordinate the Relationships of Medicine with Allied Health Professions and Services.

In the following year, 1967, the Association of Schools of Allied Health Professions—later renamed the American Society of Allied Health Professions (ASAHP)—was incorporated. Prior to that time, there was no organization that addressed the broad concerns of allied health education or provided a forum for the sharing of ideas among institutions responding to the Allied Health Professions Personnel Training Act of 1966 or acting upon the recommendations of the Allied Health Professions Education Subcommittee of 1967. At first, ASAHP concentrated on collegiate higher education: its particular concern was fostering the growth of centers of excellence built on the interdisciplinary concepts promulgated in the subcommittee report. ASAHP has since expanded its constituency to include two-year colleges and professional associations and broadened its interest to cover a wider range of concerns; however, education remains its primary focus.

Changing Times, Changing Priorities

A decade after these seminal events, when the W. K. Kellogg Foundation funded the commission study, priorities for the allied health fields had changed dramatically. Although reliable data on supply and demand are lacking at all levels—national, regional, and local—the health workforce was estimated to be over 5.1 million in 1976, and (depending on which occupations are included) the number of allied health personnel was estimated to range from 1.8 to 3 million. Consequently, the federal government has turned its attention away from manpower production and toward the problems of maldistribution, coordination of resources, and cost containment.

The emphasis on coordination and cost containment in preparing health personnel coincided with a more general pressure for austerity and control in both the education and health industries. On the education side, all but three states had established higher education boards, known commonly as "1202 commissions," to conduct "comprehensive statewide planning" in accordance with the Higher Education Amendments of 1972. On the health side, the National Health Planning and Resources Development Act of 1974 (P.L. 93-641) had introduced a host of new state and local agencies to deal with health planning and management, with particular attention to curbing rising costs of health care in the nation. At the same time that federal and state governments were emphasizing coordination and cost containment, allied health educators were coming to recognize the need for better planning and guidance to check the apparently uncontrolled proliferation of professions, specialties, and educational programs. The fear was that unless coordination could be achieved on a voluntary basis, it would almost inevitably be imposed by some part of the expanding regulatory system. Further, allied health education faced an uncertain future as more and more interested groups competed for fewer and fewer funds.

In response to a survey undertaken by the commission, allied health educators and practitioners were unified in their assessment of problems facing allied health education and services in the late 1970s (Holmstrom, Bisconti, and Kent, 1978). The most fundamental concern was the question of identity: Just what does the term *allied health* mean? If the allied health concept were more clearly defined and better understood, then the occupations encompassed by that concept might be better understood, resulting in higher visibility and greater financial support. A related concern was the proliferation and confusion of titles and terms. It was felt that unless competency requirements and responsibilities were more firmly established, such proliferation could lead only to diffusion, fragmentation, and waste of resources.

The establishment and maintenance of uniform national standards for allied health education programs and practitioners concerned many respondents, who complained that the present lack of such standards limits the horizontal, vertical, and geographic mobility of allied health personnel. Many complaints also focused on the process of accreditation, which was thought to require too much administrative effort, resulting in high financial cost, and to impede innovation.

Another frequently cited concern was the scarcity of funding for allied health relative to other health professions. Respondents felt that—on both an absolute and a comparative basis, and at the federal, state, and local levels—funding is inadequate, especially in view of the high cost of modern equipment and instrumentation for allied health education. Some program directors said they were badly in need of program improvement funds to buy new equipment and update the curriculum. Others asked how an institution could be expected to fund a high-cost curriculum adequately when enrollment restrictions limit earnings and when tuition payments are insufficient to cover costs. Other respondents were concerned about the impact of the trend toward cost containment in hospitals. In the drive to cut costs, they observed, hospital-sponsored educational programs become vulnerable, and academic institutions are increasingly expected to bear the costs of clinical training. Looking to the future, they wondered who would pay for clinical education.

Another trend frequently viewed with alarm was the upgrading of academic degree requirements for some allied health and nursing personnel. If education is increased from two to four years in certain occupations, one person asked, "who is to pay for the added cost of providing the education?"

Allied health education at the postsecondary level takes place in a wide variety of settings: hospitals; colleges, universities, and medical schools; technical, trade, and business institutes; the armed services; and federal government agencies. Given this fact—along with the proliferation of occupational titles in the allied health fields over the last decade and the general confusion of identity—it was not surprising that many respondents mentioned problems and concerns relating to the roles of different settings. Respondents from both two-year and four-year colleges believed that much wasteful program duplication exists.

Directors of programs in two-year colleges were particularly apt to express concern about the future role of their type of setting in educating allied health personnel. They felt that efforts of professional associations to upgrade academic degree requirements, as part of the process of professionalization, would depress the market value of the associate degree. Some thought that this movement would result in more education than necessary and an oversupply of baccalaureate-level graduates. They also felt that large universities received too great a share of federal funds.

Some community college administrators stressed that their institutions had a mission to serve the needs of the surrounding community. This sentiment was particularly strong among directors of two-year college programs in medically underserved areas. One commented: "Two-year colleges play a vital role, especially [in rural areas], because when local people go away to a four-year college, they don't come back."

Program directors at universities, however, defended their own type of program on the basis of quality. Some pointed out that people who act as leaders in health must have a strong background in basic sciences. Others commented that their graduates are more flexible and better able to adapt to technological change than are graduates of two-year programs.

Providing adequate clinical training to their students was a major problem for some program directors. Those in rural areas were likely to say that the scarcity of clinical facilities was the root of the problem. For others, the problem was basically financial: the high costs of affiliation with a hospital or other clinical facility and the question of who should pay the faculty. For still others, it was a question of the institution's having control of clinical training.

Lack of coordination and cooperation in allied health education was a major concern. One aspect was the need for better articulation among the various educational levels and settings and for greater standardization of curricula to facilitate transfer. Another was the need to develop core curricula and to stress interdisciplinary approaches. The question of the value of a liberal arts base also was raised, as was the question of whether what is taught today "not only reflects current practice but also stimulates . . . creative ideas for newer and better methods of health care practice."

Less imperative, but also mentioned, were concerns about continuing education (including cost, accessibility, and relevance of such programs), leadership development (especially for faculty and administrators), student selection and retention (particularly as the process discriminates against disadvantaged minorities), and, finally, research and information needs. Some respondents also emphasized that education must be related to the needs of consumers and that improved delivery systems must be developed to meet these needs.

In summary, the major problems facing allied health education and services during the late 1970s were those associated with proliferation of occupational titles and educational programs, inadequate funding, credentialing and accreditation processes, articulation, continuing education, clinical education, leadership development, student selection and retention, and research. The most persistent problem, one that is related to all others, however, was that of professional identity and self-definition, which impedes the acceptability of allied health as a concept under which diverse occupations can be brought together to work toward the common good of the nation.

The Meanings of Allied Health

Considerable confusion surrounds the term *allied health* because it is still used to describe different groups of health occupations in different settings and for different purposes. It was initially conceived as a convenient category for the purposes of clustering education and training programs other than medicine. In 1929, St. Louis University expanded its nursing school to include other health fields but did not use the term *allied health.* In the 1950s, three new schools or divisions for health occupations education were established, including the Division of Allied Health Sciences of the Indiana University School of Medicine, which was the first to use the term. Today, there are many academic units housing allied health programs, but the types of occupational programs included in these units vary from one academic institution to another, adding to the problem of identity and definition.

Some health occupations—notably physicians and dentists—have historically been excluded from the allied health category. In addition, others have been excluded by definition in federal and state laws and associated regulations; for example, federal legislation defines veterinarians, optometrists, podiatrists, and pharmacists as separate from allied health personnel. Title VII, Section 795 of the Public Health Service Act contains the following definition: "The term *allied health personnel* means individuals with training and responsibilities for (a) supporting, complementing, or supplementing the professional functions of physicians, dentists, and other health professionals in the delivery of health care to patients, or (b) assisting environmental engineers and other personnel in environmental health control and preventive medicine activities." Few people find this definition satisfactory. It is so vague that it could apply to almost any occupational category remotely connected with health. Moreover, "physicians, dentists, and *other health professionals*" is ambiguous: Is one to assume that allied health personnel are those who support, complement, or supplement the work of therapists and technologists as well as of physicians and dentists? If so, are therapists and technologists not to be considered allied health personnel? Ultimately, the definition is based on a view of health care delivery as being hierarchical in structure, with allied health workers occupying the lower levels of the pyramid. The terms "supporting, complementing, or supplementing" simply do not do justice to the wide range of services performed by allied health personnel or to the considerable autonomy with which many of them function.

The federal government's clustering of occupations for funding purposes does not help to clarify the meaning of allied health, nor does it reflect reality. For example, physician assistants programs are funded separately from programs for "associated health professions," and certain occupations that seem to qualify as both allied health and public health (for example, sanitarian) are grouped with allied health at the undergraduate level and with public health at the graduate level.

Equally confusing is the relationship of the field of nursing to allied health. On this point, the federal government has been inconsistent. For instance, the Veterans Administration defines allied health as including "all persons other than physicians, dentists, and medical or dental students engaged in providing direct services to patients" and specifically includes nursing as an allied health occupation (Administration of Veterans Affairs, 1977, p. 41). But the U.S. Department of Labor defines allied health occupations as "occupations allied to and supportive of the medical, dental, and nursing professions"; compounding the confusion, it then cites registered nurses as examples of "the highly trained allied health workers" (Bureau of Labor Statistics, 1973, p. 1). Some lists of allied health occupations exclude registered nurses but include nurse aides, nurse practitioners, and nurse midwives. Early government reports often included licensed practical nurses in the allied health group, but more recent reports generally do not.

For some purposes, the allied health occupations have been subdivided into medical allied, dental allied, and sometimes environmental allied and nursing allied. A 1974 government report using these four subdivisions included environmental engineers among the "environmental allied" (Health

Resources Administration, 1974, p. 135). Later, however, Congress specified that allied health personnel *assist* "environmental engineers and other personnel."

Perhaps the point to remember about these various definitions is that they were adopted by the federal government strictly for funding purposes. In a sense, then, they are mere expedients; they should not be accepted as the final word on what the term *allied health* comprises.

Views of Professional Associations. As an aid in clarifying the meaning of the term *allied health,* the following question was included in the commission's thorough survey of professional membership associations: "What does the term *allied health* mean to you? Is it useful? Can it be improved?" In addition, the questionnaire asked whether the responding association considered itself an allied health association. Of the seventy-nine responding associations, 57 percent regard themselves as allied health associations; just 22 percent think that allied health is a useful descriptive label as it now stands; many respondents feel that current usage of the term is inaccurate or misleading. What allied health really means, or what it should mean, according to their comments, is *a horizontal alliance, the joining together of health professionals working toward a common goal: the best possible total patient care.* According to some, physicians, nurses, and all other health personnel who work together should be considered allied health. Others see allied health personnel as colleagues of the physician or dentist. In either case, the emphasis is on the consumer of health services rather than the provider, as the following comments illustrate:

> Allied health education should mean all professions allied in health: medicine, nursing, dentistry, OT, PT, and so on.
>
> There are three terms which designate the relationship of health professionals to medicine: "Paramedical" implies secondary or accessory to medicine. "Associate" means partner in a more formal relationship. "Allied" expresses more the joining of equals for common purposes. "Allied

> health" is preferred. . . . Allied health implies the team concept, giving services whenever a special demand is to be met, in a collaborative undertaking. Allied health means cooperation among health organizations in mutual support and recognition of the common objective to provide quality care to health consumers. "Allied health" implies working with other professionals in the total care of the patient. This brings the total team together—including physician, surgeon, dentist. "Allied health" is a more inclusive term. It reaches into the total field of professional education. Previous designation was "ancillary," which had a tendency to downgrade the practitioner.
>
> "Allied health" is a group of medically-oriented professions providing distinctive health care services to the public. Although each profession is an entity unto itself, the commonality of health care delivery participation unites the group toward a common goal, the highest quality patient care possible.
>
> "Allied health" [implies a] genuine concerted effort to work harmoniously, to work for the well-being of the consumer, and to come together as separate specialists with a prevailing sense of dedication and mutual respect. Moreover, this concept must extend itself into each city, medical complex, and corridor where any given care-giver applies health care skills. If the spirit of "allied health" is reduced to exposure only at infrequent gatherings, then the ultimate purpose and worth of health care is proportionately reduced. "Allied health" must be a full-time working concept.

Some respondents indicate that the horizontal alliance concept is appropriate, but that allied health is not usually used in this sense. Because the term impedes professional recognition, they believe that it should be discarded in favor of some other term such as *health profession, health care profession,* or *health-related profession.* For example:

> "Allied" should mean joined or united. As it has been applied to "health" it has been interpreted to include all those other than medical professions. With the acceptance of the team approach to health care any terminology that is exclusive seems outmoded. Many of the health care professions have been recognized as providers of primary care although they are not members of the medical profession. We suggest for your consideration "health care professions" or "providers of health care."
>
> "Allied health" is the designation of a concept implying a team approach to health care. However, this generalized idea has had difficulty in being accepted as have the many professions so designated. Because identity and status are so important to all professionals, it would be desirable to drop the "allied" and speak only of health professions.

Other respondents take a more traditional view, interpreting "allied" to mean *allied vertically to the physician or dentist.* According to this view, allied health personnel are those who work under the supervision of the physician or dentist, providing *supportive services.* Some professional associations representing personnel whose acknowledged role is supportive find this meaning acceptable:

> "Allied health" refers to those groups or individuals who are directly involved in patient care under the supervision and/or direction of the physician. [Name of association] prefers being considered an "allied health" association since [name of personnel represented] do fit the concept described above.

Others find this traditional use of the term demeaning and indicate that they would prefer some other designation:

> "Allied health" as we have heard it used refers to secondary personnel whose function is to

> assist the primary care practitioners. We much prefer the term "health practitioner."

Respondents who dissociate themselves entirely from allied health are more inclined than others to view the personnel covered by this term as relatively low-level assistants or aides.

Conclusions of the Commission. The commission endorses the following definition of *allied health personnel*: "all health personnel working toward the common goal of providing the best possible services in patient care and health promotion." In a dynamic field, multiple tasks and occupations are essential if the common good is to be so advanced. So extensive is the body of knowledge required for good health care today that no one person could know or do all the things to provide optimal care for one other person. Thus the effective delivery of health services, now and in the future, depends on an appreciation of the significant contributions of each member of the health team.

The term *allied health* is useful in indicating the alliances that need to be built for effective health care delivery and promotion. As a concept, it implies much more than a mere collection of occupations but conveys a collaborative approach to providing health services. For practical purposes, it has been and can continue to be used with some flexibility, depending on particular purposes and circumstances. For government funding purposes, it is an easy way of grouping all health occupations not already covered in separate legislation. For academe, it is a convenient way of grouping all health disciplines not already organized in separate schools. As the nation works to achieve its health goals through education, research, and practice, the commission hopes that this concept of allied health can attract the broadest possible constituency.

Construed narrowly, the term *allied health education* refers to the formal preparation of a sizable segment of the health workforce, the composition of which may vary depending on the occupations included as allied health. This formal preparation can take place in a collegiate as well as noncollegiate setting; it can involve short-term as well as long-term training; it can lead to a certificate or a graduate degree; and it can range from basic occupational preparation to advanced education to various continuing education activities that keep professional competencies current.

As a concept, allied health education too has much wider implications. In 1966, when the term *allied health education* was first introduced into federal legislation, it implied a certain amount of collaboration and coordination to meet the major health manpower goal of the day: an increased supply of practitioners. It implied an emphasis on the health care system as a whole over the interest of particular occupations or specialties. And it described the formalization of preparation for health careers, the move away from ad hoc or on-the-job training toward more rigorous and, at the same time, more broadly based academic education.

These same implications are valid today, but the context has changed. Since 1966, we have witnessed rapid social, economic, and political change in this country. We have moved from a period of affluence, expansion, and optimism into a period of financial stringency, more intense competition for resources, and a growing emphasis on accountability—conditions that impose difficult demands and offer new challenges for allied health education. Communication, cooperation, and collaboration—desirable in an era of boundless resources—have become absolutely necessary in an era characterized by public intolerance of waste. Placing the public's need for good health care above the ambitions of specific occupations is no longer just an admirable goal; it is essential for survival. And even though much good has resulted from the increased formalization of allied health education, the question now arises as to whether this trend is really in the best interest of the health care system and the public it serves.

Ten years ago, the mandate for allied health education was relatively simple: to increase the supply of health personnel. Now the emphasis must shift from quantitative to qualitative goals, which are considerably more complex. The national focus in the 1980s should be on the quality of health services and on the effectiveness and efficiency of modes of preparing health personnel to deliver these services. The survival and growth of health services has always depended on the public belief that these services contribute to the well-being of the individual. If this public trust is to be maintained, programs in allied health education must be shown to be related to practice needs, which include as the highest priority the improvement of personal well-being. The recommendations in this report embody this new emphasis. Whatever the time and effort required to shift thinking at the national and local levels from manpower numbers to quality issues, they are necessary if commitment and support are to be won for the initiatives required to move ahead.

II

Current Status of Allied Health Occupations and Manpower

The allied health occupations, which compose a major segment of the total health workforce, include a broad range of services, the contributions of many of which are not fully appreciated by the public. The competitive activities of professional associations representing various allied health occupations are sometimes said to exacerbate this situation. Yet many professional associations, having established their identity, are now willing to work together to create a stronger image and voice for allied health occupations. This chapter describes characteristics of allied health occupations, showing areas of commonality and similarity in roles and functions, and presents the viewpoints of professional associations regarding their current concerns and attitudes toward building new alliances.

Characteristics of Allied Health Occupations

According to the latest figures available (1976), the allied health occupations—excluding nursing and related services—comprise over 1.8 million health workers, about 36 percent of the entire health workforce of 5.1 million. As a group, they are outnumbered only by personnel in the nursing occupations: Nurses and nurse auxiliaries constitute 49 percent of the health workforce. Physicians, osteopaths, dentists, veterinarians, optometrists, podiatrists, and pharmacists together account for only 13 percent. A few occupations not classified in any of these groups, such as clinical psychologist and chiropractor, make up the remaining 2 percent.

The total number of allied health workers varies, of course, depending on the particular occupations included. If the one million nurse aides are considered allied health personnel (as they often have been), and if clinical psychologists are added (as they have been to the federal government's list of allied health personnel), then the total number jumps to nearly 3 million, and the proportionate representation to 57 percent.

The allied health occupations are extremely heterogeneous and personnel work at various levels. Available manpower estimates, which use broad occupational titles, do not provide accurate information on numbers of allied health personnel at different levels. Tentatively, anywhere from 565,000 to 727,000 allied health personnel work as technologists, therapists, administrators, and other relatively high-level positions. From 450,000 to 515,000 people work as technicians, 280,000 to 468,000 as assistants, and 340,000 to 350,000 as aides. Some occupations are numerically strong (for example, in 1976, there were 130,000 medical laboratory technologists, over 80,000 medical laboratory technicians, 140,000 dental assistants, 30,000 dental hygienists, 48,000 dietitians and nutritionists, 24,000 physical therapists, and 43,000 medical and psychiatric social workers), but others involve rather small numbers of personnel (in 1976, there were just 4,000 biomedical engineers, 500 health economists, 1,400 medical writers, 3,000 medical librarians, 800 to 1,000 optometric technicians, 1,100 art therapists, and 2,200 music therapists).

Because of the large number of occupations and the small membership of some of them, the public is generally unaware of the extent to which allied health personnel contribute to patient care and health promotion. Nor does the public understand that allied health occupations differ considerably in the competencies and the amount of education required to perform their services effectively. This lack of public recognition has serious consequences, namely, inadequate federal support and peripheral legislative attention, particularly when compared to medicine and nursing.

Services Provided by Allied Health Personnel. Several attempts have been made to describe allied health occupations by grouping them according to the kinds of services they provide. One such grouping, mentioned earlier, separated the occupations into medical allied and dental allied. Such a scheme, which may have been meaningful when the number of occupations and the range of functions was less extensive, has little value today. It reflects the historical development of some occupations, as well as their service links to physicians and dentists, but fails to indicate how allied health personnel serve the patient or client.

The 1967 status report by the Allied Health Professions Education Subcommittee of the National Advisory Health Council proposed a simple classification of occupations based on service orientation: patient oriented, laboratory oriented, administration oriented, community oriented, and other (Bureau of Health Manpower, 1967). In a somewhat different approach, Weiss (1966) divided health occupations into two major groups, each with subgroups called "job families": patient-care oriented (mental, nursing, medical, and dental) and technical oriented (technical and laboratory, administration and planning, data processing, environmental, and health research). Yet another classification scheme was based on service goals or types of care: for example, preventive, crisis, rehabilitative, and long-term care (Broski and others, 1977).

The commission's classification of health services (see Figure 1), which reflects these different approaches, was developed to indicate how allied health personnel function within the health system and why it takes many different occupations to meet today's health service needs. Personnel in a single occupation may perform many of the services described in this scheme, but probably could not perform all.

The scheme has two major components: (1) institutional, direct "patient" care services, and (2) community health promotion and protection services. Within the patient-care component, services are described chronologically in terms of what happens to the patient from the time care is sought, through evaluation and diagnosis, to treatment. Of course, a patient will receive care from different types of health personnel, depending on the setting, the problem, and the course of treatment.

Among those who provide services at the time of patient entry are such allied health personnel as ambulance attendants, emergency/disaster specialists, emergency medical technicians, and emergency rescue technicians, as well as physician assistants and other primary-care generalists. The reception/administration function is likely to be handled by a medical or dental secretary, a medical office assistant, or some other administrative worker.

Allied health personnel are involved in evaluation and diagnosis in a variety of ways. Initial assessment of the problem may be the responsibility of physician assistants, dental hygienists, mental health technologists, or medical social workers. Assessment is also an integral part of the treatment provided later by physical therapists, occupational therapists, speech pathologists, dietitians, and others. A further aspect of evaluation and diagnosis is the testing conducted by laboratory personnel, who may have no direct contact with the patient but who provide necessary information for treating the patient's problem. Another essential element in diagnosis may be the tests conducted with medical equipment by radiologic technologists, ultrasound technical specialists, nuclear medicine personnel, cardiology equipment personnel, and others who do come into contact with the patient.

Figure 1. Health Services Classification Scheme

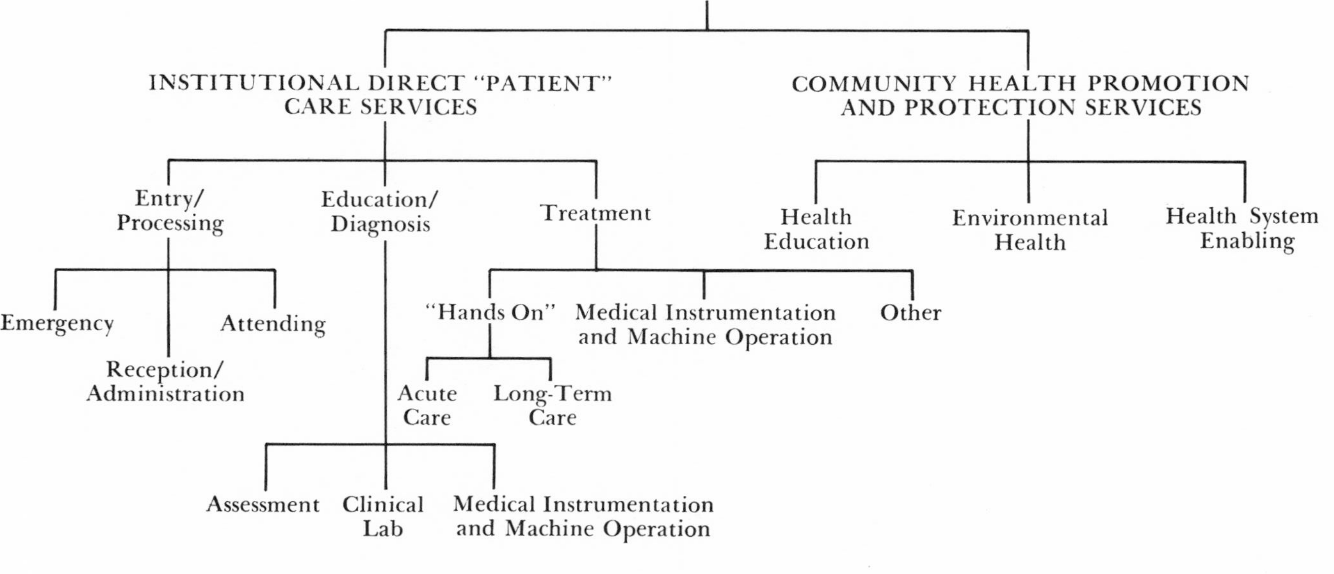

A wide range of therapeutic services is provided by allied health personnel: "hands on" care, medical instrumentation and machine operation, administration of medication, and management of the patient's diet. "Hands on" services may involve either acute care provided by operating room technicians, obstetrical technicians, and surgeon's assistants or long-term care provided by personnel in occupational therapy, physical therapy, mental health, social services, counseling, speech and hearing, and other therapies. Among the people who operate therapeutic instruments and equipment or who work with therapeutic devices are radiation therapy and respiratory therapy personnel, dialysis technicians, cardiopulmonary technicians, ophthalmic dispensers, dental laboratory technicians, and a variety of other specialists.

The second component of allied health services relates to community health promotion and protection. Both in health care facilities and in the community, allied health personnel work to maintain and improve the general health of the public through education, elimination or control of environmental hazards, management of health systems, and research and development. The allied health occupations that engage in community health promotion and protection services include nutritionists, hygienists, population and family planning specialists, health educators, school health educators, and those who store and communicate health information (for example, medical librarians, medical illustrators, and health writers). Some environmental health personnel are oriented primarily toward community health (for example, sanitarians, environmental health technicians, sanitarian aides, environmental engineers, and environmental engineering assistants) and apply different types of expertise to problems involving the quality of air, water, food, and other features of the environment. Other environmental health personnel, such as health physicists and health care facilities housekeepers, are concerned with eliminating hazards from health care facilities. Still others, such as industrial hygienists, focus on health in the workplace.

Concerned with maintaining and improving health care delivery systems are administrators of health care facilities, health planners, medical records personnel, medical computer specialists, and other health systems specialists. Finally, many allied health personnel work to promote the general health of the public through research and development. Biomedical engineering personnel develop new instruments, equipment, and processes for health care; other allied health statisticians and scientists (for example, biostatisticians, epidemiologists, toxicologists, and public health scientists) seek to discover the causes of disease and to establish safe levels of exposure to chemical compounds.

Knowledge and Skill Requirements. The health sector as a whole probably requires a greater range of knowledge and skills than any other industry in our society. Allied health occupations differ with respect to the types of competencies they require: all the way from the performance of routine tasks to the generation of new knowledge through research. Similarly, as Chapter Four indicates, the range of educational preparation is very broad, varying from little or no postsecondary education to postdoctoral study. The time required for such preparation ranges from a few weeks to many years. Educational level and preparation time, however, are not necessarily related. The amount of time that a given student has to spend in an occupational program should depend on the knowledge and the skills base which that student brings to the program and the intensity of his or her study.

Allied health occupations also differ with respect to the scientific foundation of their knowledge base. For example, medical laboratory personnel must have a firm grounding in the biological and chemical sciences; social services and counseling personnel require preparation in the social sciences; whereas occupational therapy personnel draw upon both physical and social sciences, as well as the humanities.

Some allied health occupations are based in an established health discipline, such as physical and occupational therapy (see Table 1). The knowledge base—while founded on natural sciences, social sciences, humanities, or some combination thereof—is specifically related to health service. The skills and techniques are applicable principally to health. In other

Table 1. Type of Knowledge and Skill Base of Allied Health Occupations, by Range of Levels Within Disciplines

Range of Levels Within the Discipline	*Primary Knowledge Base for Allied Health Occupations*	
	Single Health Discipline	*Nonhealth Discipline or Multiple Disciplines*
Broad range of levels	Clinical laboratory services Dietetic and nutritional services Occupational therapy Physical therapy Radiological services Respiratory therapy services Speech and hearing services	Rehabilitation—other (for example, art therapy, music therapy) Social services and counseling Environmental health Biomedical engineering Health administration and planning Medical records
Narrow range of levels	Dental services Physician assistant Vision care Emergency services Medical instrumentation and machine operation Nuclear medicine services Pharmacy services Podiatric services Veterinary services	Medical assisting Health education Information and communication Clerical office work

allied health occupations, the knowledge and skills learned in a nonhealth discipline or in multiple disciplines are applied to health problems. For example, biomedical and environmental engineers bring their engineering knowledge and techniques to bear on health problems: the former by developing new instruments and devices, the latter by attempting to control environmental hazards, particularly pollution. Medical librarians could presumably function in any library setting but have developed additional specialized knowledge. Art, dance, and music therapists apply nonhealth principles and techniques to the rehabilitation of physically and mentally ill patients.

As further illustrated in Table 1, some occupational areas include more than one knowledge level—for example, occupational therapy includes occupational therapist and occupational therapy assistant. Some of these multilevel disciplines (for example, medical laboratory technology) have evolved with some degree of knowledge and skill progression; in others, however, a smooth knowledge and skill progression has not developed. Different levels are considered separate occupations, and complementary educational programs have not yet been developed. This lack of continuity in education results in dead-end careers for many.

Range of Unsupervised Action. Another dimension on which allied health occupations vary greatly is degree of autonomy: the type and amount of independent or unsupervised action expected or permitted. Many allied health personnel are closely supervised by physicians, dentists, or other practitioners, whereas a large number of others are not. Generally, the scope of unsupervised action is greater for allied health personnel involved in community health promotion and protection services than for those in institutional, direct "patient" care. Even in the latter, however, some occupations have a long history of autonomy in service delivery (for example, social workers, speech pathologists and audiologists), whereas others have expanded their autonomy considerably in recent years. Physical therapists have operated on a fee-for-service basis in the United States for well over fifty years, and an increasing proportion of practitioners are now working on this basis. Further, in California, patients may seek care directly from physical therapy clinics without referral by a physician. In certain situations, such as in underserved areas, physician assistants provide primary health care under periodic physician review. Increasingly, other allied health personnel are taking on responsibility for unsupervised patient care services to meet health care needs.

In addition, many allied health personnel are responsible for supervising the more routine activities of technicians, assistants, and aides. Medical technologists supervise medical laboratory technicians and assistants; sanitarians supervise environmental health technicians and sanitarian aides; and physical therapists supervise physical therapy assistants and aides.

Common Grounds

In the past decade or so, the rapid and somewhat erratic growth of allied health education programs has paralleled the rapid growth and fragmentation of the allied health occupations in response to a variety of stimuli: advances in technology (for example, in respiratory therapy and nuclear medicine), national concern with particular health problems (for example, polio, drug addiction), and the desire of some occupational groups to delegate their more routine tasks to others. As various levels and new titles evolved and eventually became recognized as separate entities, the number of occupations multiplied. For instance, in the medical laboratory field alone, one finds medical technologists, medical laboratory technicians, clinical laboratory assistants, specialists in blood bank technology, chemistry technologists, hematology technologists, histologic technicians, medical laboratory scientists, microbiology technologists, and public health laboratory scientists, among others.

Whatever the historical causes of this proliferation, the results have all too often included conflict, competition, and confusion. Occupational groups have tended to isolate themselves; mutual appreciation has been replaced by hostility and mistrust, and self-interest has overshadowed the need for collaboration in working toward the common good.

Role of the Professional Associations. The organizational development of different health occupations reflects the fragmentation of the field. The professional associations represent personnel with varying levels of status or identity in the health care delivery system. Some professional organizations are new, others have a long history; some represent large constituencies, others relatively small ones; some have considerable influence, others do not. They are at different stages of development, and not all of them follow the same pattern. Nonetheless, broad similarities can be identified.

The staff survey of professional associations, supplemented by informal interviews and discussions, revealed widespread interest in collaboration, mixed with some suspicion and anxiety. At present, the health-related occupations seem to be reaching out to others and, at the same time, to be concerned with preserving their own identity, improving their quality, and building their knowledge base.

Because of the heterogeneity of the allied health occupations and the tendency of occupational groups to isolate themselves, communication and cooperation in developing the content and processes for the education of allied health personnel have been limited. Professional association representatives, in response to the commission's survey, acknowledged that each discipline has tended to develop independently, going its own way "rather than building on what other disciplines have learned." Respondents emphasized that communication and cooperation should start with the "determination and recognition of commonalities and differences."

Commonalities Perceived by Professional Groups. As a starting point in identifying commonalities, the commission sought the opinions of the professional associations themselves. In developing the questionnaire for the survey mentioned previously, the staff compiled a list of all the occupational titles included in the ASAHP *Glossary*—adding physicians, dentists, psychologists, nurses, and other health occupations—and asked respondents to review this list and to indicate: (1) "all occupations you consider closely related to the occupations represented by your association" and (2) "the three occupations that you consider most closely related to the occupations represented by your association." Respondents were also asked to give their reasons for choosing the three "most closely related" occupations. The common grounds mentioned by professional associations were as follows:

Similarities in Knowledge and Work Content

- functions; techniques
- curricula
- service areas; objectives
- equipment; instruments
- client population
- work setting
- health-relatedness
- part of the body

Ties Through Job or Career Relationships

- collaboration; teamwork on the job
- supervision patterns (association personnel supervise or are supervised by the same personnel; both occupations have same supervision or backup person)
- area of career change

- patient-client-provider relationship

Parallels in the Development or Status of the Occupation

- level of training
- type of occupation (for example, new specialties)
- credentialing
- privileges and responsibilities; autonomy

Professional Association Activities

- collaboration; joint membership

The reasons most frequently mentioned by professional association representatives for naming other occupations as closely related to their own were that the occupations were similar in functions or in curricula. In addition, common work situations and relationships, as well as historical development patterns and status, were often cited as reasons for linking occupations with dissimilar—although, in some cases, complementary—functions and curricula.

An analysis of the responses to the questions about commonalities resulted in the identification of three clusters of health occupations (see Table 2).

- *Cluster one:* primary care (medical, dental, nursing, vision care) and related personnel
- *Cluster two:* health promotion, rehabilitation, and administration personnel
- *Cluster three:* test- and measurement-oriented personnel

Cluster one: The commonalities mentioned by fourteen professional associations produced a cluster of occupations that were characterized by their primary care (or direct support of primary care) and related functions. Central to this cluster were nurses, physician assistants, and dental auxiliary personnel; each of these groups perceived its commonalities with the two others. Further, medical assistants—as well as pharmacy, vision care, podiatric, and respiratory therapy personnel—were linked with at least two of the three central occupational groups. Almost all the occupations in this broad cluster were seen by their professional associations as working closely with physicians or dentists.

Table 2. Clusters of Allied Health Occupations Based on Commonalities Perceived by Professional Associations Responding to the NCAHE Survey

Cluster I	*Cluster II*	*Cluster III*
Primary Care and Related Personnel	*Health Promotion, Rehabilitation and Administration Personnel*	*Test- and Measurement-Oriented Personnel*
Nurse midwife	Dietitian	Biomedical engineer
Ambulatory nursing administrator	Health planner	Biomedical technician
Physician assistant	Sanitarian	Ultrasound technical specialist
Medical assistant (also medical/dental business manager, secretary, medical insurance clerk, allied health educator)	Environmental health technician	Nuclear medicine technician/technologist
Podiatric assistant	Sanitarian aide	Medical physicist
Hospital pharmacist	Environmental engineer	Health physicist
Hospital pharmacy technician	Health care facilities housekeeper	Health physics technician
Dental hygienist	Medical communications specialist	Radiologic technologist/technician
Dental assistant	Medical illustrator	Radiation therapy technologist/technician
Optometric assistant/technician	Medical photographer	Diagnostic medical sonographer
Ophthalmic dispenser	Medical librarian	Medical radiation dosimetrist
Ophthalmic laboratory technician	Health educator	Nephrology nurse
Orthoptist	School health educator	Nephrology technician
Ophthalmic assistant/technician	Teacher of the deaf	Cardiopulmonary technician
Respiratory therapist	Teacher of the visually handicapped	Chemistry technologist
Respiratory therapy technician	Physical therapist	Cytotechnologist
	Physical therapy assistant	Histologic technician
	Rehabilitation counselor	Medical laboratory assistant
	Alcohol/drug abuse specialist	Medical laboratory scientist
	Occupational therapist	Medical laboratory technician
	Occupational therapy assistant	Medical technologist
	Recreational therapist	Public health laboratory scientist
	Music therapist	
	Art therapist	
	Manual arts therapist	
	Rehabilitation therapist	
	Population and family planning specialist	

Some linkages were made between occupations in this cluster and those in Cluster Two. For instance, the associations representing dietetic and nutrition personnel and health planning personnel (all occupations in Cluster Two) linked their members with physician assistants and nurses. Almost no close linkages were perceived between the occupations in Cluster One and those in Cluster Three; the single exception was respiratory therapy, which was located in Cluster One but was seen to have commonalities with test- and measurement-oriented occupations.

Cluster two: The responses of twenty-seven professional associations indicated that a complex network of relationships exists among occupations whose emphasis is health promotion, rehabilitation, or administration. Medical information, communications, and records personnel were associated with each other as well as with planning and education personnel. Medical records personnel were also linked with people in administration and physical therapy. Dietetic personnel were associated primarily with education, planning, administration, and environmental health personnel, and this last group in turn was associated with planning. Commonalities were perceived among occupational, physical, and other therapies, and between these occupations and mental health, social services, counseling, education, planning, and administration.

Several occupations in this cluster were associated with physicians, clinical psychologists, speech and hearing personnel, and nurse specialists. Other linkages were made with physician assistants, dentists, public health workers, and biomedical engineers.

Cluster three: Personnel in the testing- and measurement-oriented cluster were linked together by their professional associations on the basis of teamwork and collaboration on the job, as well as overlap in knowledge base and job functions. In some cases, the "most closely related" occupational groups were those who worked in some way with the same equipment. Biomedical engineering, health physics, radiologic, and nuclear engineering personnel were seen as interrelated. Clinical laboratory personnel were linked closely with medical instrumentation personnel, who in turn were linked closely with biomedical engineering and nuclear medicine personnel.

This group of occupations also indicated commonalities

with physicians and with a variety of other health personnel, including allied health educators, environmental personnel, and health planning and analysis personnel.

Collaboration Among Professional Associations. The territoriality and isolationism of individual professional groups is widely acknowledged and almost universally deplored; what is less often recognized and discussed is their growing willingness to collaborate. The commission's survey questionnaire asked professional association representatives to indicate in which of eight listed areas they were currently collaborating "with other associations representing allied, associated, or independent health professions" and in which areas collaboration would be beneficial. Their responses indicate the extent of current collaboration:

- developing the professions, 48 percent
- formulating policy on credentialing and other matters, 46 percent
- planning educational programs, 41 percent
- increasing public awareness of the professions, 39 percent
- promoting legislation, 39 percent
- designing curricula (interdisciplinary, core, and so on), 37 percent
- supporting research and innovation, 32 percent
- working on state and regional plans for the future utilization and education of health personnel, 19 percent

The potential for future collaboration is great; at least two thirds of the association representatives said that collaboration would be beneficial in each of these eight areas. The willingness to collaborate with other professional organizations in matters relating to education is especially significant, as it is an essential ingredient for successful implementation of a number of the commission recommendations in Chapter Six.

Several umbrella organizations serve as vehicles for general-purpose communication among allied health occupations. The National Health Council, whose constituency includes all organizations involved in health care, acts as a clearinghouse for information, especially on careers. The American Society of Allied Health Professions (ASAHP) is the only organization that provides a forum for addressing problems of broad concern to all those involved with allied health education and services. A primary objective of this organization is to facilitate communication, cooperation, and collaboration both among the professions and between the professions and educational institutions.

The Coalition of Independent Health Professions, an umbrella organization for associations that represent personnel who may practice without direct physician and dentist supervision and who usually have the baccalaureate or higher degree, facilitates general-purpose communication among a specific segment of the health fields and is more practice oriented than education oriented.

Response to the commission survey shows that some associations take issue with the "unified voice" concept promulgated by ASAHP several years ago, when it was generally acknowledged that the fragmentation of allied health fields weakened efforts to present a persuasive case to Congress on matters affecting the education and utilization of personnel in these fields. This concept was enunciated in a 1972 address by Merlin DuVal, then Assistant Secretary for Health and Scientific Affairs, Department of Health, Education, and Welfare: "Who can say what it is that the allied health professions want to do, which are the directions in which they choose to move, what it is they wish to recommend to Congress to help the professions improve the quantity and quality of service to the American public? . . . If you speak with a multiplicity of voices and concerns, little will be heard, and even less will be heeded. At best, the result will be confusion; at worst, it will be inefficiency" (DuVal, 1972, p. 13).

The comment of one respondent to the commission survey epitomizes the concern of some associations: "Being perceived as allied with other groups where the training of practitioners takes place on a lower academic level (for example, B.A. or below) may exacerbate difficulties in obtaining appropriate recognition for services." Another respondent points out that her association is "autonomous from all other professional organizations and must speak for its membership on all issues affecting the practice, education, recognition, legislation, and economics" of the profession. Some express the opinion that collaboration can be reconciled with the drive for independence if such efforts focus on problem solving, particularly with respect to educational matters.

In summary, some collaboration is already taking place among professional associations representing allied health occupations, and most association spokespersons believe that further collaboration would be beneficial. Others express some reservation about identifying too closely with other (usually lower-level) occupations and would prefer collaboration only in specific problem areas. One good example of the successful use of a topic-focused approach such as is endorsed by many professional associations was an ASAHP-sponsored National Conference on Continuing Education, held in September 1978, that attracted many new people who came from a variety of backgrounds but shared a common interest in resolving some basic questions about continuing education in the health fields.

Concerns of Professional Associations

The commission's survey questionnaire also asked professional association representatives to comment on "the greatest needs" of allied health occupations today. Their responses reflect some of the same concerns as were voiced by respondents to the "grass roots" survey (see Chapter One), though on some matters, the emphasis is different.

Identity. Like the allied health program directors, the representatives of professional groups are most concerned about identity, status, and recognition. More specifically, they mention the need for higher salaries, more responsibility, independence from the American Medical Association, and reimbursement for services.

There are several reasons why many allied health fields have difficulty winning appropriate recognition and support. First, they may be relatively new, having emerged recently in response to changing health service needs. Medicine, dentistry, and nursing have a long history, but the majority of health occupations titles were unknown before 1940. Because they grew out of the older established health professions, the newer occupations tend to be viewed as subservient, even though some of them have developed a comprehensive knowledge base and include practitioners who hold doctoral degrees. Second, some occupational titles are difficult for the layman to comprehend. Pathologists and radiologists are also physicians; cytotechnologists and ultrasound technical specialists have no umbrella title to shelter under, except "allied health," which means different things to different people. Finally, the allied health occupations as a group constitute a very large component of the total health workforce, but single allied health occupations may not be numerically large.

The lack of recognition suffered by many health occupations has several consequences. One is that some occupational categories receive very little financial support for education, training, and research. For example, of the federal funds distributed to academic institutions through the Bureau of Health Manpower over the last decade, only about 4 percent went to allied health fields, whereas 45 percent went to medicine and osteopathy, and 21 percent went to nursing. Another consequence is that the educational programs of these occupations have relatively low status in the very types of academic institutions (for example, research universities, health science centers) that could play the greatest role in developing future leaders and contributing to their knowledge base for education and practice. Further, the earnings potential in these fields is still relatively low. Although wages of allied health manpower rose rapidly during the last twenty years (Fuchs, 1976), the increases in earnings over time are still less substantial for allied health personnel than for other workers with comparable educational levels.

The most obvious response to the problems of identity and recognition has been the drive to upgrade credentials, both academic and professional. Many allied health occupations have raised the degree levels required for practice, and further upgrading is on the agenda of several associations. So far, the contention that these increased levels of education are necessary to perform the work in question can neither be proved nor refuted by the available evidence (Galambos, 1979). Practitioners, educators, and association representatives in some of these occupations have admitted in informal discussions that a major reason for the upgrading is the desire for recognition, including higher salaries. The typical rationale is that occupation X performs work on the same level as occupation Y, but occupation Y is better paid because it requires a baccalaureate for entry; therefore, occupation X wants to deny entry to anyone with less than the baccalaureate and may even be considering basic occupational programs at the master's level.

Professional credentialing–including program accreditation and the certification, registration, and licensure of practitioners–serves both as a "quality assurance" mechanism and as a mechanism to encourage or enforce the upward trends in educational requirements. Such credentialing also helps to upgrade professional status by limiting access to jobs, thus creating a favorable job market. The deep concern for identity manifested by the representatives of professional associations suggests that pressures to upgrade the educational requirements for entry into allied health occupations will continue and that professional controls over educational content through certification and accreditation mechanisms will increase.

Quality Assurance. In fact, another major concern of professional associations is quality assurance. Some respondents to the survey speak in general terms of the need to assure that practitioners are qualified to perform the roles and functions of their occupations. Others speak of the need for national standards and for a coordination of the credentialing process. Some perceived "needs" reveal that different health professional associations held diametrically opposed views, with some insisting on mandatory credentialing to assure quality of practitioners, and others favoring alternatives to mandatory credentialing and a reduction in "guild" control.

The controversial topic of accreditation has involved both professional societies and educational institutions in joint study and activity. Most noteworthy are the Study on Accreditation of Selected Health Education Programs (SASHEP) and the American Medical Association's (AMA) Committee on Allied Health Education and Accreditation (CAHEA). Currently, CAHEA plays a major role in allied health accreditation. The evolution of this role parallels the evolution of the allied health professions as a whole. As was pointed out in Chapter One, the AMA has collaborated with professional associations in accrediting educational programs for almost fifty years. Until 1976, the Council on Medical Education had primary responsibility in this area, whereas the current structure gives the collaborating professions a stronger voice.

Appointed by the AMA Board of Trustees, the members of CAHEA—five physicians, four allied health professionals, a hospital administrator, a dean of a university school of allied health, a student or recent graduate, and two representatives of the public—are chosen for their "broad interest and competence in the fields of the allied health professions and services" (American Medical Association, 1978b). CAHEA is currently chaired by an allied health dean. The collaborating professional associations and the Council on Medical Education "carry equal weight in the adoption of the *Essentials,*" which may be developed by either group. In addition, CAHEA utilizes a Panel of Consultants, including representatives of thirty-three health organizations, to formulate procedure statements. These statements address such key issues as the accreditation of experimental or innovative programs and the fragmentation and proliferation of accrediting bodies.

CAHEA has not, however, won unanimous support. A number of associations object to the involvement of the AMA, a point that was made by some association representatives either in interviews or in response to the commission survey. As an extreme case in point, the American Physical Therapy Association (APTA) House of Delegates voted in 1976 to sever its ties with the AMA and to conduct accreditation independently. Because physical therapy program accreditation continued under CAHEA as well, programs became subject to quality assessment by two bodies.

With respect to certification, a new collaborative venture

—the National Commission for Health Certifying Agencies (NCHCA)—is being watched closely. The NCHCA, with ASAHP surving as secretariat, was formally organized in December 1977 as a result of the recommendations of a government report, *Credentialing Health Manpower* (Public Health Service, 1977, p. 7), which proposed that

> a broadly representative national (nonfederal) certification commission . . . be established to perform the following functions for allied health occupations:
> 1. Develop and continually evaluate criteria and policies for the purpose of recognizing certification organizations and monitoring their adherence to these criteria.
> 2. Participate in the development of national standards.
> 3. Provide consultation and technical assistance to certification organizations.

The NCHCA was formed to address such problems as the lack of certification for some occupations; competition among certifying agencies for other occupations; variation in requirements (from very specific standards to no requirements other than payment of a fee); dilution of standards due to liberal grandfather clauses; inadequate disciplinary procedures; and the diversity of standards between licensure boards and certification agencies, a diversity that affects the quality of health services and creates obstacles for both geographic and career mobility. By providing competitive agencies with the opportunity to meet and discuss the issues, the NCHCA hopes to effect some consensus on standards and procedures. Moreover, NCHCA promotes changes in certification processes by the criteria it establishes for membership. Of particular significance is the criterion that certifying bodies establish alternative routes to eligibility for certification other than formal education in order to qualify for membership by 1982.

Communication, Cooperation, and Collaboration. The professional associations also express major concern about communication, cooperation, and collaboration. One respondent to the survey mentions the need to develop "an attitude of mutual respect and reduce competition, recognizing each other's expertise and finding ways to complement one another." Joint planning—including the development of mutual objectives and the formulation of coordinated action to "counter common threats"—is suggested.

Historically, the drive for status by individual occupations has often frustrated attempts at collaboration, just as the quality-assurance mechanisms, imposed partly to enhance and protect professional status, have impeded interdisciplinary approaches to education. Some associations find, however, that membership in umbrella organizations can be an effective way of working on problems related to professional status. Some respondents report that they joined the National Health Council for "prestige" and the Coalition of Independent Health Professions for "strengthening efforts." A member of the American Society of Allied Health Professions (ASAHP) comments:

> We have encouraged [name of association] to belong and participate fully in ASAHP because it has been our only vehicle for real involvement with other health professions and professionals outside [the field]; our "window-on-the-West." It has raised our level of awareness concerning problems and trends within the entire health field. It has increased our perceived power and balance of power within [the field]. It has provided us with an opportunity to stand up and be counted in addressing issues that affect our professional future in a meaningful way. We are leaders and peers here, which has not been the case within the [field] community. It has also given us a focus in dealing with government at the federal level.

Government Relations. The professional associations responding to the commission survey generally agree that their government relations activities must be improved. Both separate efforts by individual associations and collaborative efforts involving a number of associations are seen as essential. Professional associations must represent their own concerns but, at the same time, may speak to legislators more effectively, when dealing with broader issues that concern them all, if they join forces. Many respondents acknowledge that ASAHP can play a vital role in working with professional associations and other groups such as the Coalition for Health Funding and the National Health Council to develop and convey to legislators the consensus of the field.

Education and Research Needs. Finally, professional association representatives mention a number of concerns relating to education and research, most of which are addressed in the commission's recommendations (Chapter Six). In the area of education, they cite the need to improve quality, make education more relevant to practice, develop interdisciplinary approaches and core curricula, promote continuing education, and foster leadership development.

Respondents believe that research is needed to clarify roles and functions, identify practice needs, make services more effective and cost-beneficial, establish a firmer scientific base for particular occupations (for example, nutrition), and devise methods for identifying and measuring professional competencies. These education and research needs are related in two ways: First, some of the research topics mentioned must be addressed if education needs are to be met; second, educational settings are particularly favorable locations for developing the expertise needed to meet the research needs of the health fields.

The Rallying Point

The commission feels that the term *allied health* is valuable, not so much as a label for this extraordinarily heterogeneous and constantly changing group of occupations but as a concept. Given the vast range of health service needs that exists today, the term *allied health* is best used to mean a patient- or client-focused alliance involving all health practitioners. It is this meaning that can serve as a rallying point, marking the beginning of a new collaboration in education as well as in service.

If this concept is to work—if the public is to understand that allied health implies many diverse practitioners with different educational backgrounds, skills, and functions who work together for the purpose of serving the patient or client—then a conscious and concerted effort must be made to change the negative image of the allied health practitioner as a low-level worker serving the physician. Unfortunately, this image—which has led some of the more influential occupational groups to dissociate themselves entirely from allied health and to adopt an adversary stance toward organized medicine—is deeply entrenched.

Largely responsible for perpetuating this negative image is the federal government's definition of allied health personnel quoted earlier, which is echoed in other major documents. For instance, one publication of the American Medical Association describes the development of allied health occupations as follows (Committee on Allied Health Education and Accreditation, 1978, p. 73):

> Historically, new allied health occupations developed in these steps: identification by a physician of a need for a new helping role; the training by that physician of a person to fill that role; the increase in numbers of the new type of personnel to the point where an organization is formed to speak for them; and, finally, the establishment of informal and then formal collaboration with the appropriate medical specialty groups and the AMA Council on Medical Education in the adoption of *Essentials* for the education of such personnel. Education and training for occupations that began at the physician's side has, over the years, grown roots back into colleges and universities.

This description may have had some validity many years ago, when allied health occupations were known as allied medical or paramedical occupations, but it does not hold true today for the majority of such occupations. As this chapter has indicated, allied health personnel serve many functions beyond simply helping the physician. Some have little or no contact with physicians, others play roles that are better termed collaborative than supportive, and still others have themselves spawned new occupations.

In the past, it may have been possible for one person to know all there was to know about health care and to provide all the necessary services. But that possibility ended with the information explosion and the resulting specialization in knowledge and skills. Today, health care and health promotion may best be conceived as a giant jigsaw puzzle made up of many different but tightly interlocking pieces, each playing a significant part in making up the total picture. Allied health leaders must take responsibility for communicating this concept to the public, not through exhortation but through example. Greater public awareness of the contributions made by all health occupations will result in a stronger identity for each.

III

Outlook for Allied Health Careers

To make predictions about future patterns of health service delivery, one must take into account the complex relationships among a number of factors: demographic, socioeconomic, and political trends; government policies; legal decisions; reimbursement patterns; credentialing, unionization, and the policies of professional associations; technological changes; disease trends; patterns of utilization of services, people, and settings; and the supply-demand balance for various categories of manpower. Although crystal gazing is always an uncertain business, the emerging picture indicates that this nation is involved in a revolution in the health care delivery system. This revolution was triggered by general social trends, changes in national policies and priorities, and changes internal to the health care delivery system itself, and it will culminate in a changed environment for health service delivery in the last two decades of this century. Within this environment, allied health personnel are likely to play an increasingly important role as the value of their services is more widely recognized.

Influences on Demand

The rapid growth of the allied health occupations in this country paralleled an equally rapid growth in the demand for many types of health services. Between 1967 and 1977, hospitals reported that inpatient visits rose by 26 percent and outpatient visits by 78 percent (American Hospital Association, 1978, p. v). The rate of surgery increased by 24 percent between 1965 and 1975. In the four years between 1971 and 1975, emergency room visits per person per year actually doubled. Increased use can also be seen in long-term facilities, emergency mental health services, and dental services (National Center for Health Statistics, 1977, pp. 258-282).

Factors leading to the increased use of health care services include population growth, changes in private insurance coverage, and the intensifying role of the federal government to provide better access to health care for the poor and the aged. Today major differences in the amount of utilization of health services between the poor and the nonpoor that existed a decade ago seem to have diminished (Fuchs, 1979). The growth in the utilization rate and the broadening of the types of services offered have also resulted in an increased demand for allied health personnel.

Although the use of health services in general will almost certainly continue to increase in the future, the Commission's Advisory Panel on Health Service Needs concluded that *the demand for health services will increase at a decreasing rate.* This conclusion was based on careful consideration of the various forces and counterforces described next.

General Social Trends. The demand for health services will undoubtedly be affected by the sheer size of the population in future years. In 1960, the population of the United States numbered 180 million; the estimate for 1980 is 225 million, and for 1990, over 250 million. However, the changing characteristics of the population may be even more important in determining demand than the expanding size.

The U.S. population is aging: Between now and the year 2000, the over-65 age group will have grown by 40 percent, and the 45 to 64 age group by 50 percent. This trend is attributable both to demographic factors and to advances in health care. It will become even more pronounced if, in the face of a continuing energy crisis, reduced highway speed limits are strictly enforced and automobile accident rates drop further. This aging trend has been called "a built-in 'time bomb' for medical care spending" in that the incidence of chronic disease, more associated with the aged than the young, is bound to rise (Wynder and Kristein, 1977, p. 1507).

An anticipated baby boom in the 1990s will accompany the aging trend to produce a situation that would demand increased attention to the health care needs of the very young and the very old. The school health movement will almost certainly increase in strength as the numbers of preschool and school-age children rise dramatically.

The demand for health services will be further increased by certain socioeconomic trends already long established and likely to continue: As the nation's citizens become more educated, urbanized, and affluent, they expect more services; as the consumer movement grows, they demand better services.

Health-related behavior patterns must also be regarded as important factors. Such self-destructive behaviors as drug abuse and alcoholism show no sign of abating, so demand for health services relating to these problems is likely to increase. More positive factors contributing to this increased demand are greater public acceptance of the ideas that alcoholism and drug abuse are illnesses and, concomitantly, greater willingness on the part of victims to seek treatment. Similarly, less stigma is attached these days to seeking help for mental illness. Apparently, rehabilitation programs of all sorts are filled to capacity almost as soon as they are initiated or expanded.

There is growing evidence that in the United States today, health is no longer significantly related to income, except perhaps among the very poorest segment of society. Health is, however, still closely related to education: that is, to a great extent it depends on the ability of better-educated people to delay gratification and to change or curb their unhealthy behavior and, to a lesser extent, on the availability of health care (Fuchs, 1979). Recent years have seen the public becoming slowly but definitely more health conscious, paying greater attention to the formation of good personal health habits. Such changes highlight the growing importance of preventive medicine and health promotion, both of which require allied health services.

Disease Prevention and Health Education. As is becoming more widely recognized, the health status of the nation's citizens could be greatly improved if more emphasis were placed on keeping people well in the first place and on reducing or eliminating health hazards. Section 1502 of the National Health Planning and Resources Development Act of 1974 (P.L. 93-641) names the following as two of ten national health priorities:

> The promotion of activities for the prevention of disease, including studies of nutritional and environmental factors affecting health and the provision of preventive health care services.
>
> The development of effective methods of educating the general public concerning proper personal (including preventive) health care and methods for effective use of available services.

Moreover, the Public Health Service's *Forward Plan for Health: 1977-1981* emphasizes the significant role of behavior modification and environmental science in health care delivery. Alcoholism, smoking, and speeding behind the wheel are cited as phenomena having "profound health implications" that are determined by social, economic, cultural, and psychological factors (Public Health Service, 1975). The report calls for greater attention to the relationship between affluent, sedentary lifestyles and cancer, cardiovascular disease, and other chronic illness, and also calls for broadscale action to limit environmental hazards. Currently, the federal government is spending only a penny or two of each health dollar on prevention, although private foundations are supporting demonstration and evaluation projects related to preventive approaches.

Would the overall demand for health services be increased or reduced by a new national emphasis on prevention and behavior modification? Though that question cannot be answered with any certainty, it is safe to say that such an emphasis would certainly alter the nature of health services. The preventive orientation involves a shift from episodic care to more continuous or comprehensive care. Traditionally, the physician responded to each complaint as it arose; with the new approach, care is given as needed to preserve and protect well-being. Wynder and Kristein (1977, p. 1507) point out that "if we begin to work now on reducing preventable chronic illness, for example, lung cancer, cancer of the upper alimentary tract, chronic bronchitis, coronary heart disease, cirrhosis of the liver, and emphysema, we could be saving many billions of dollars per year in five to ten years," and health services would shift from acute care (which is expensive) to preventive care.

Ironically, controversy over implementing preventive approaches centers on their costs rather than their benefits to personal welfare. Proponents have not always come up with convincing evidence for the cost-effectiveness of this approach. Another obstacle, related to the first, is the long-term nature of the impact of any preventive program; long-term benefits are often not salient for political purposes. Moreover, the goals of a preventive program may conflict with the desires or preferences of the population at which it is directed, with individual rights at stake.

The available evidence suggests that preventive approaches are most likely to be implemented when grass-roots involvement is assured. In the future, planning groups such as Health Systems Agencies (HSAs) may help to promote preventive services by working with local groups to identify community needs, providing necessary support systems, and acting as liaison and mediator between the community and state and federal agencies.

Improved Access to Health Care. According to Section 1502 of the National Health Planning and Resources Development Act of 1974, the nation's number one health priority is the provision of primary health care services to medically underserved areas. Many federal, state, and private initiatives address the needs of the medically underserved population, which numbers an estimated 49 million—about 27 million in rural areas and 22 million in urban areas (United States Senate Committee on Human Resources, 1978). For instance, the Department of Health, Education, and Welfare supports the Rural and Urban Health Initiatives (including Community Health Centers), Migrant Health Programs, and Primary Care Research and Demonstration (formerly the Health Underserved Rural Areas Program). The state of North Carolina has established seventeen rural primary care centers staffed by family nurse practitioners and physician assistants under the supervision of physicians. In addition, private foundations, such as the Robert Wood Johnson Foundation and the W. K. Kellogg Foundation, have funded major programs aimed at improving access to health care.

Although many different forms of delivery have been tried, the most promising seem to be primary health centers, group health practices, and comprehensive health centers. The basic staff usually consists of physician assistants or nurse practitioners and personnel who can perform some laboratory work; dental and preventive services personnel are often included (Davis and Marshall, 1977). Recently, because of cost constraints, the trend has been to cut back on services in these programs, but this trend is beginning to be reversed. Federal agencies are now placing renewed emphasis on the provision of preventive services and on community outreach, both of which rely heavily on allied health personnel.

One possible model for the future is the mini-health care system, in which physicians based in towns of 50,000 or less work together as a group to address the problems of underserved areas, going into outlying areas on a rotating basis, while other health personnel serve in permanent outpost positions.

Expanded Concept of Health. The concept of health has come to mean much more than physical well-being; it has already been expanded to cover mental health and, in the future, it may well have a social component. Certainly this social component is emphasized in the statement from the *Forward Plan for Health* cited earlier. Its implementation, or integration into the health care system will depend, to a large degree, on the economy of the nation.

The Commission's Advisory Panel on Health Service Needs expects that the demand for mental health services will increase substantially and that the way such services are delivered will change radically. Those trends are already under way: Over the past twenty years, the volume of treatment episodes in organized mental health settings has quadrupled, and mental health services are shifting from inpatient facilities to other settings. The current tendency is to remove patients from inpatient psychiatric facilities as quickly as possible, either by releasing them or by transferring them to foster homes, group homes, or general hospitals with psychiatric beds (National Center for Health Statistics, 1978, p. 70).

Although the tradition in this country has been to separate mental health care from general health care, the need to integrate the two has become more widely recognized, and steps have been taken to effect such an integration in the provision of primary care. For example, one pilot program includes mental health personnel in clinics run by the federal government. If successful, the model may be implemented on a larger scale. One likely result of this integration would be an increase in the demand for mental health care services: first, because the stigma attached to seeking such services would be reduced; second, because broader insurance coverage for such services would be assured.

Already the health care system has begun to address social problems related to drug abuse, alcoholism, family planning, and aging. Thus the line of demarcation between the health care system and the social services system is beginning to blur. As concern over society's ills—as opposed to the individual's illnesses—mounts, the health care system may become more directly involved in dealing with other problems such as crime, juvenile delinquency, and the disintegration of the family.

Reimbursement Patterns. Reimbursement is a major factor in the demand for health care services. It stands to reason that people are more willing to use services if the costs are covered by a third party, and the evidence bears this out: For example, Medicare-Medicaid legislation led to an estimated 10 to 15 percent increase in the demand for ambulatory services (Newhouse, Phelps, and Schwarts, 1974, p. 46). Reimbursement patterns affect not only overall demand but also the types of services that are used. In fact, consumer overuse of hospital services has been blamed largely on third party payment mechanisms, which tend to provide more extensive coverage of inpatient than outpatient services.

This situation may change, however, as third party payers give more emphasis to the appropriate utilization of services, chiefly by expanding coverage for and actively supporting a wider range of services in a wider range of settings. Such an expansion may also further cost-containment efforts. Blue Cross and Blue Shield plans have invested over $30 million in developing and operating Health Maintenance Organizations (HMOs), which emphasize prevention and early detection of disease and the use of ambulatory services, chiefly through their organization and provider payment incentives. The plans also seek to limit hospitalization by supporting a second opinion prior to surgery, ambulatory surgery, preadmission testing, and home health care. Blue Shield has initiated a Medical Necessity Program to stop routine payment for procedures judged to be of unproven value, of questionable usefulness, or redundant. Thus the new emphasis is on widening the range of services—including noninstitutional services—and on helping the consumer to make more appropriate use of these services. This emphasis is consistent with federal priorities for national health, as listed in Section 1502 of the National Health Planning and Resources Development Act of 1974.

Coverage of dental services is expected to increase dramatically in the near future as many more workers participate in prepaid dental plans. The number covered is expected to rise from 9 million in 1975 to an estimated 68.6 million by 1990, and inclusion of dependents should raise total coverage from 16 million to 107 million (Kriesberg and others, 1978, p. vi).

After years of controversy, it seems likely that some form

of national health insurance will be in place by 1990, and that a comprehensive health insurance plan will become a reality by the year 2000. The commission's advisory panel predicts the following scenario: The federal program will be phased in, at first simply filling existing gaps and later rounding out health coverage and making it more uniform. The federal program will be additive; that is, it will not eliminate what private groups have already achieved in health insurance.

According to this scenario, a national health insurance program will have only limited impact on the demand for health services, which—as was mentioned earlier—is expected to increase at a decreasing rate, but it will alter the configuration of health services. Specifically, more services (some of them substitutive for existing inpatient services) will be provided in an ambulatory setting; incentives and constraints will be introduced to decrease the use of inpatient services; and the needs of the elderly for custodial care in an institutional setting will become a matter of growing social concern. Increased services in ambulatory settings, in organized settings generally, and in institutional settings for the elderly will mean a net increase in the demand for some allied health services.

The future of inpatient services under national health insurance (and the demand for allied health personnel to provide such services) will depend on the outcome of several conflicting trends. As ambulatory services are broadened, more diseases requiring treatment are likely to be discovered, and so initially the use of inpatient facilities will increase. Over the longer term, however, cost considerations will probably lead to incentives and constraints designed to reduce the use of inpatient services (especially in surgical, diagnostic, and clinical areas) and to increase the types of services provided in ambulatory settings.

The impact of national health insurance on the utilization of allied health manpower will depend in large part on what services in the ambulatory settings are covered and on methods of reimbursement. Thus the nature of the financing and the kinds of benefits provided—rather than simply the increase in funding—will be extremely important, and decisions on these matters will probably be made on the basis of cost considerations.

Whatever the accuracy of the advisory panel's prediction that a national health insurance plan will be in operation by 1990, a trend already exists to cover services provided through expanded functions of allied health personnel. Recently, under the Rural Health Clinic Services Act of 1977 (P.L. 95-210), Medicare payments have been allowed for services performed by physician extenders in rural health clinics, operating under only periodic physician review and consultation.

Generally, third party payers base their reimbursement on the cost of the service (which is usually determined by the current norm) rather than on the type of health worker who provides the service. Thus there has been no incentive to use lower-cost personnel. With the growing emphasis on cost containment, however, third party payers may decide to reimburse at the level of the least costly practitioner qualified to perform a particular service, thus encouraging greater use of lower-salaried personnel. One plan that already follows this policy is that of the International Retail Clerks Union. Whether pressures to use allied health personnel to save costs are counterbalanced by physician oversupply in certain geographical areas remains to be seen.

New Technology. The consensus of the Advisory Panel on Health Service Needs is that total expenditures for new technology will increase at a decreasing rate and that, despite the Certificate of Need Program, the health care providers will continue to invest heavily in new technology. In 1976, hospitals spent an estimated $730 million on labor-saving devices (Tracka, 1977, p. 50), but data from the Stanford Research Institute show that the tendency is now to order larger quantities of less expensive equipment for many services. According to a spokesman from Stanford Research Institute, during the past four years, expenditures for CAT-scanning equipment have dropped from about $100 million to $20 million, whereas expenditures for ultrasound equipment have risen from about $30,000 to $100 million. The reasons for this shift from CAT-scanning equipment to ultrasound equipment are several: first, body scans are not reimbursable; second, ultrasonic devices are less expensive; third, ultrasonic devices require fewer and less-trained personnel to operate than do CAT-scanners. Thus, although labor-saving devices are being ordered, and in a wider range of settings, the net effect is probably to increase the use of radiology personnel, though not necessarily in hospitals.

Data from the Stanford Research Institute also show that, in 1976, hospitals spent $122 million on automated wet-chemical analyzers, which reduced the need for laboratory personnel. Nonetheless, despite this increasing automation in the clinical laboratory, the overall number of personnel has not declined because service intensity has quadrupled as insurers recognize more tests. Hospitals are, however, becoming more likely to use independent commercial laboratories than to do their own in-house testing, since Medicare will pay only in the lowest quartile of usual and customary costs for laboratory tests.

Even though the introduction of labor-saving devices may eventually reduce the overall demand for technical specialists, it seems clear that new technologies will continue to be introduced, rendering some kinds of skills obsolete but creating new demands for others. Some allied health occupations are more closely involved with technology than others and thus more susceptible to obsolescence as technologies change, unless they have skills that are easily transferable. New technologies will, however, affect all areas of practice and all practitioners, regardless of whether their primary function is related to specific equipment or machines.

Employment Patterns

The hospital is the predominant employer for personnel delivering certain allied health services (for example, clinical laboratory, dietetics, radiology, rehabilitation, respiratory therapy). However, about two thirds of all allied health personnel, including some in those occupations referred to above, work in other settings such as ambulatory facilities, nursing homes, laboratories, and private group practices. Although the employment of allied health personnel is bound to be influenced by trends in hospital services and staffing patterns, the greatest growth areas in the future can be expected to be in nonhospital sites.

Employment in Hospitals. In 1976, hospitals employed over 3 million full-time-equivalent (FTE) workers, though differences in occupational titles make it difficult to enumerate accurately the types of allied health personnel involved. According to unpublished data from a 1976 national survey of hospital employees, at least one in five FTE hospital employees was an allied health worker; this figure does not include nurse aides or orderlies. Studies comparing staffing patterns in 1968 and in the early 1970s indicate substantial increases for certain categories of allied health personnel. One study of the Boston area hospitals indicated that, between 1968 and 1973, the number of physicians increased by 28 percent and the number of registered nurses by 25 percent, but gains were even greater for certain allied health occupations: radiologic technicians, 210 percent; physician assistants, 175 percent; respiratory therapists, 92 percent; operating room technicians, 60 percent; speech therapists, 53 percent; and medical technologists, 49 percent (Goldstein and Horowitz, 1977, p. 72).

Similarly, studies conducted in Pennsylvania showed the following increases between 1968 and 1974: radiation therapy technologists/technicians, 326 percent; respiratory therapists, 234 percent; certified medical librarians, 135 percent; occupational therapy assistants, 134 percent; certified medical records technicians, 119 percent; certified histologic technicians, 92 percent; and social workers, assistants, and aides, 70 percent. Further, in Pennsylvania, higher-level allied health personnel such as technologists and therapists played an increasingly significant role; only one in four of the higher-level occupations suffered losses, compared with three in five allied health occupations at the aide or assistant level (Pennsylvania Department of Education, 1977).

The Commission's Advisory Panel on Health Service Needs predicts that even though more services are likely to be provided outside of hospitals, the demand for hospitalization will rise in the near future, primarily because of the anticipated 50 percent increase between now and the year 2000 in the over-64 age group, which has a hospitalization rate three-and-a-half times the national average. The panel believes that the effects on hospitalization rates of any increased spending for prevention would not be felt for at least twenty years, but pressures on the part of third party payers for noninstitutional care might have an impact within the next ten years. The immediate outlook, then, is for an overall increase in the numbers of allied health personnel employed in hospital settings.

The increase will not, however, be uniform for all allied health occupations. Some categories may be affected by the voluntary efforts that some hospitals have initiated to curb rising health care costs by improving the efficiency of their operations. These efforts include the introduction of cost-saving technology (for example, Centrex system, computerized pharmacy), establishment of multihospital corporations, sharing of resources, group purchasing, and improvement of management controls (for example, preventive maintenance, zero-based budgeting, inventory control, product standardization). But the main approach to cost containment involves people; hospitals are trying to increase productivity by changing utilization patterns and to cut back on personnel costs by reducing staff and introducing labor-saving devices.

The commission found, from review of literature and interviews with hospital administrators and others, that several types of personnel are particularly vulnerable to staff reduction efforts: those in relatively low-level positions (for example, assistants, aides), those in positions not directly involved in patient care (for example, maids and porters), those performing services for which hospitals can contract out (for example, computer services, medical illustration), those involved in community-oriented services (for example, health educators and nutritionists), and narrowly trained technicians. Cutbacks may result from attrition, planned elimination, and consolidation of positions. In some cases, specialized functions are being absorbed by persons with broader preparation, especially registered nurses. The advisory panel believes that the demand for certain types of technicians in the future will be influenced by the market for registered nurses.

Cost-containment efforts have also affected the number of services for which hospitals contract out or which they share with other facilities. According to a recent survey of hospitals conducted by the American Hospital Association, more than four in five hospitals now share at least one service with another facility, an increase of 20 percent since 1975 ("AHA Survey Finds Hospitals . . . ," 1978, p. 4). The most commonly shared services in 1978 were purchasing, electronic data processing, blood banking, laboratory services, education and training, laundry/linen, biomedical engineering, credit union, and diagnostic radiology. These patterns suggest that cost-containment efforts may increase the demand for office workers, medical records personnel, and administrators and for generalists with broad skills who can help expand the services of physicians, while at the same time depressing the demand for narrow-skilled technicians, assistants and aides, and personnel whose services are not specifically patient centered.

Employment in Ambulatory Settings. Recent years have witnessed an increase in the number of nonhospital-based ambulatory facilities—such as neighborhood health centers, health maintenance organizations (HMOs), and clinics—where allied health personnel account for a large proportion of staff. In the Boston area, for instance, 54 percent of the staff employed in ambulatory settings in 1973 were allied health practitioners: mostly social workers, medical technologists, and radiology personnel (Goldstein and Horowitz, 1977, p. 77).

Generally, the public does not object to being treated by nonphysicians. Using data from a household survey conducted by the National Opinion Research Center (NORC) in 1975, the Center for Health Administration Studies at the University of Chicago ran some special cross-tabulations for the commission. Over four in five respondents in this survey said they would be willing to let a nurse or doctor assistant do the preliminaries of a medical examination (for example, taking medical history, taking blood pressure), and almost three in five said they would allow such personnel to provide follow-up care and treatment after a physician had carried out the diagnosis and prescribed treatment. A Rand Corporation study in 1974 came to the following conclusions (Newhouse, Phelps, and Schwarts, 1974, pp. 21-22):

> The supply of ambulatory services could, over the long term, be expanded whether by an in-

> crease in physician productivity (that is, more services rendered per physician hour) or by the allocation of more resources to the ambulatory sector. An increase in productivity, some believe, might best be achieved by widespread introduction of HMOs. However, although HMOs may have the potential to enhance productivity, there is no evidence that this potential has been realized in the delivery of ambulatory care. Other mechanisms designed to influence physician productivity, such as peer review, may ultimately prove to be effective in the ambulatory sector, but their value has not yet been demonstrated.
>
> A far more promising approach to the problem of productivity is likely to be through the expanded use of allied health personnel. The more widespread use of aides and physician assistants in ambulatory care offers a potentially highly effective way of delivering each unit of service at a cost less than at present.

One recent study estimates that the proportion of the population enrolled in HMOs—only 2 percent in 1979—may rise to between 6 and 28 percent by 1990. The effect of such an expansion would be to increase the demand for allied health personnel in administration, medical records, clinical laboratory, and dental services (Swift, Montalvo, and Ward, 1974).

The commission's advisory panel believes that ambulatory care of all kinds will increase in the future, especially if national health insurance covers the services provided in the ambulatory setting, and that physicians will be increasingly likely to locate in "organized" settings, including group practices. Further, as services are broadened, ancillary services added, and task delegation becomes more common in these settings, more openings for allied health personnel will become available, especially for those who have more generalized training (including "multicompetency" personnel—that is, those who can function in more than one occupational role).

Employment in Long-Term Care Facilities. The nursing home industry has grown tremendously in the last two decades.

Between 1960 and 1976, the number of nursing homes in the United States increased by 140 percent (from 9,582 to 23,000), the number of nursing home beds by 301 percent (from 331,000 to 1,327,358), the number of employees by 550 percent (from 100,000 to 650,000), and the number of patients by 245 percent (from 290,000 to 1,000,000). Most dramatic was the increase of 2,000 percent in revenues received by the industry (from $500 million in 1960 to $10.5 billion in 1976). Since the number of senior citizens increased by only 23 percent over this same period, these phenomenal growth rates cannot be attributed entirely to the increase in this population (Moss and Halamandaris, 1977, p. 7). Other influential factors are better insurance coverage (including Medicare and Medicaid) and such social trends as greater participation of women in the labor force and the greater mobility of the U.S. population, which makes it difficult to care for the aged within the family. Thus, as Fuchs (1979, p. 11) points out: "A considerable amount of what we think of as an *increase* in health care is not an increase at all, but a substitute for care that was formerly provided within the family."

The need for well-trained personnel to care for the aged and handicapped—whether in nursing homes or at home—is critical. In 1976, about 80 to 90 percent of the medical care in nursing homes was provided by aides and orderlies, who have relatively little training. As more Medicare and Medicaid funds go to nursing homes, and as the public becomes more aware of the growing role that nursing homes have in taking care of the aged, the federal government can be expected to exercise greater controls over the nursing home industry, tightening standards and causing an upgrading of both the facilities and the personnel.

Also likely to lead to increased demand for well-trained allied health personnel is the increasing federal emphasis on alternatives to institutional care for the aged and handicapped. Families can be assisted in caring for the aged and handicapped at home by the provision of home health services, such as part-time or intermittent nursing care; physical, occupational, or speech therapy; and other medical and social services, including homemaker-home health aide. The last is a fast-growing occupation: According to information provided by the National Council for Homemaker-Home Health Aide, Inc., in 1962, there were about 300 homemaker-home health aide programs in forty-four states; today there are about 3,700 such programs in fifty states and Puerto Rico. Nonetheless, the current supply of such personnel (around 85,000) falls far short of the estimated need (300,000), and with an increasingly aging population, the demand is certain to grow.

Another alternative to long-term institutional care is the adult day care center, where health, social, and nutritional services are provided to people sufficiently ambulatory to be transported between their homes and the center each day. These centers, which currently number around 200, utilize a number of allied health services, including rehabilitation, nutrition, and recreational therapy. These alternatives to long-term institutional care in an institution will almost certainly gain in popularity, especially since they seem to be cost-effective (National Center for Health Statistics, 1978, p. 104).

Reinhardt (1979, p. 283) argues that "the Medicare system will increasingly come to be looked upon as support for the general long-term 'social care' of the aged—as distinct from 'health care' proper." Already noninstitutionalized forms of long-term care, as well as recent moves to improve institutionalized care, have opened up new vistas for allied health services. In addition to the traditional nursing and medical care, new modes of service are being utilized, including rehabilitation, social counseling and therapy, nutrition, and health education. Persons trained in geriatrics and gerontology will also be increasingly in demand, both in institutional and noninstitutional settings.

Another area that has implications for allied health practitioners is the care of the dying in hospices. Hospice is a specialized health care program that provides personal support emphasizing the management of pain for the terminally ill and their families. Most care is centered in the home. Currently, there are just over 100 hospices in the United States; over 200 are in the planning stage. Most hospices are directed by a physician, who is supported by a staff of other physicians as well as nurses, social workers, physical therapists, and others. The hospice movement has every likelihood of becoming stronger. Moreover, learning how to deal with death and how to meet the needs of the dying and their families has become, or should become, an essential ingredient of training for the health professions.

Employment in Business and Industry. The demand for allied health personnel in business and industrial settings is on the increase and can be expected to intensify. Employers are concerned about their rising health costs, which have doubled in the past three years. In 1977, business and industry accounted for over $34 billion, or 21 percent, of the nation's total health care expenditures, through insurance programs. These expenses —plus the amounts spent on Workmen's Compensation, disability, sick leave, and other programs—comes to about $1,000 per year per employee (Ellwood, McClure, and Rosala, 1978).

In an effort to cut these costs, many business organizations have established on-site health programs, ranging from small nursing stations to large primary care clinics. A study conducted several years ago (Smith, 1976, p. 33) showed that 25 million workers in companies with over 500 employees have access to such in-house services, which tend to utilize a wide variety of allied health personnel. Expanded on-site health care programs use medical assistants, dental hygienists, therapists of various kinds, and laboratory and radiology personnel. Industrial prevention and health promotion programs use health educators, nutritionists, counselors, and therapists. Programs directed at special illnesses draw upon mental health aides, counselors, alcohol and drug abuse specialists, social workers, therapists, and rehabilitation personnel. Safety programs involve health physicists and other environmental specialists.

According to the commission's advisory panel, once an on-the-job health program has been established, it tends to grow, especially if it proves to be cost-effective. Thus it is likely that business and industry will expand such programs in the future, by starting laboratories, setting up stress-testing apparatus, and developing fitness and hypertension control programs. It seems reasonable to assume that all these efforts would require the services of allied health personnel.

Overall Prospects. Most authorities agree that, nationally, the demand for allied health personnel will continue to rise over the next decade, although the period of rapid expansion has ended. As the commission's Advisory Panel on Health Service Needs concluded: "The demand for allied health personnel will increase, but at a decreasing rate." The Bureau of Labor Statistics (1978) assesses the employment outlook for allied health occupations as favorable, citing the following factors:

- population growth and the aging trend
- a more health-conscious public with greater interest in rehabilitation, speech and hearing, and other specific services
- the increasing number of patient services and diagnostic tests
- the growth in the number of group practices, HMOs, and nursing homes
- increased insurance coverage and ability to pay
- greater awareness and acceptance of allied health personnel because of changes in medical and dental education and the demonstrated effectiveness of these personnel
- the growing complexity of management and information systems

Nonetheless, the bureau sounded some cautionary notes: Though prospects are favorable for speech and hearing occupations, competition will be keener, and increased emphasis will be placed on having a master's degree. The demand for both radiologic technology and occupational therapy personnel will rise considerably, but if the output of educational programs continues at the same rate as it has in the past, the result could be an oversupply of graduates.

Respondents to the commission's survey of professional associations were equally optimistic when asked to rate, for their member occupations, job prospects now and ten years in the future. Current or future prospects were rated as "not so good" or "bad" for just a handful of occupations, including some related to education and communications and several categories of technicians and aides. However, the regional and local picture with respect to demand may differ considerably from the national picture. In some states, the distribution of health personnel can be expected to remain uneven, with inner-city and rural areas continuing to experience shortages while other areas are characterized by a surplus.

Because of the considerable variation in demand from one community to another, close scrutiny of the local situation is essential. Institutions that prepare graduates primarily for local employment will need to keep tuned to the changing demand in their area by maintaining close contact with employers and by using market study techniques. If better manpower information at the state and regional levels could be provided regularly to higher education institutions, they might do a more effective job of assuring that their output of graduates in particular fields neither exceeds nor falls short of the demand. Difficulties in attracting students, placing graduates in jobs, and arranging clinical affiliations should be regarded as signs that a program may be losing its viability.

Implications for Education

Some broad implications for allied health education can be drawn from this discussion of trends and probable future needs in health services and settings. Educators and administrators in allied health programs would be wise to give greater attention to building flexibility and adaptability to changing requirements, exposing students to varied practice environments, and orienting students to comprehensive care.

Building Flexibility and Adaptability. Generally, the more broadly prepared the practitioner, the more likely that practitioner will be to find employment in health. As is well documented, small hospitals and other health care facilities need personnel trained in primary care; few can attract or afford full-time staff members who are highly specialized. In some cases, they may provide a range of services by sharing personnel or by drawing personnel from long distances on a part-time basis, but they nonetheless need a core staff with a wide range of competencies to provide basic services in such areas as laboratory, x-ray, and respiratory therapy. According to the AHA report, *Delivering Health Care in Rural America* (1977b, p. 20): "In small rural hospitals, staff members frequently need to 'double up' in their roles. On a given day the obstetrics ward might be empty, but more nurses might be needed in cardiac intensive care. Perhaps one person could direct the medical record department and the medical library; another might logically serve as both a laboratory worker and an x-ray technician."

Although highly specialized and narrowly educated personnel continue to be utilized in large urban hospitals, recent experience with cost-containment efforts indicates that these people are particularly vulnerable to cutbacks. Some technician positions are being absorbed by more broadly trained personnel, notably registered nurses. Generic programs with core content, rather than discrete and highly specialized programs, will enable graduates to accommodate more easily to new technological developments. Such adaptability is particularly important for those occupations that require relatively lengthy preparation. The longer the time interval between the initiation of an educational program and the production of graduates, the greater the risk that highly specialized skills and techniques learned in the program will have become obsolete. Further, the greater the investment in education that turns out to be obsolete, the greater the waste of time, money, and talent.

Coupled with the need for generic preparation will be an increasing need for continuing education and other short-term retraining programs that will allow practitioners to update their skills and knowledge and to adjust to new technologies as well as to other changing health service demands. In 1973, Pellegrino (1974) discussed the applicability of the concept *confluence* to allied health. *Confluence* is "a joining of the diverse streams of functions and tasks, now partitioned among so many technical or professional specialties" (p. 83). He suggested that ASAHP should develop "a set of generic functions, reducing the number of categories of workers performing those functions and consolidating the educational preparation for each" (p. 83). Pellegrino argued that the development of and education for generic functions would provide the practitioner with a base upon which to build future changes of functions resulting from new developments. Further, this would free allied health professionals from the entrapment within too narrowly defined fields that have a tendency to produce dead-end jobs.

In 1973, this was perhaps beyond the capabilities of the field. Today technology and know-how exist to move toward "confluence"; many research studies have documented the overlap between professions. Task analyses and role delineation methodologies have been developed and utilized by a number of occupations to describe the practice needs of their professions. The results of some of these have been translated into educational content. What is needed now is for the professions to work together to identify commonalities in roles and functions that can be translated into educational content of a more generic nature. Ultimately, clusters of occupational groups might develop a knowledge and skill foundation upon which specialty training could be built. Such a foundation would enable practitioners to adjust to changing health care needs with a minimum of retooling. It would ensure that even with the approaching obsolescence of particular specialty areas, a major component of the investment in learning would not be wasted.

Exposing Students to Varied Practice Environments. At present, the most common clinical affiliation site for most allied health programs is the hospital. With the growing emphasis on ambulatory care, it is important that students be exposed to a wider variety of clinical settings, such as neighborhood health centers, health maintenance organizations, and on-site health facilities in business and industry. Further, a better integration of didactic and clinical education might allow students a wider choice of shorter-term practicum in a number of clinical sites as opposed to a longer experience in one setting. Efforts should also be increased to provide various combinations of teamwork in clinical training, leading to a better understanding of the interplay of roles and functions of different health practitioners in different settings.

Orienting Students to Comprehensive Care. Emerging trends and patterns, as well as national priorities enunciated in federal legislation, point to the need for an educational approach that orients students to comprehensive care. The expanded concept of health care, the new emphasis on prevention and on healthy life-styles, the growth of "new" health care centers, the broadening of insurance coverage, the increased incidence of socially related disorders, and the aging of the population, all these forces suggest that, if they are to deliver services effectively in the future, health practitioners of all types must be concerned with the whole patient or client. Developing such a concern calls for a shift away from emphasis on acute care or episodic care. The comprehensive care approach requires an awareness of behavioral and environmental factors that may pose risks to the individual's continued well-being. Such an approach also requires greater attention to human values and a greater appreciation of the impact of illness on the patient and the patient's family.

An Opportunity for Leadership

At the beginning of this chapter, it was stated that this nation is experiencing a revolution within the health care delivery system. Regardless of whether the rapid changes described here are considered revolutionary or not, there is little doubt that the priorities, settings, services, and personnel utilization patterns of tomorrow will not be the same as today.

Allied health personnel can make a significant difference in national efforts to increase access to health care while holding down costs. The services they provide are relevant to both traditional health care and new concerns such as disease prevention, mental and social health, health promotion, problems related to aging and to alcoholism and drug abuse. They are also relevant to new settings such as rural clinics, health maintenance organizations, and hospices. Allied health personnel can assume leadership in planning and management of integrated health services to achieve the goals of quality service and cost-effectiveness. They can assume leadership in clinical practice to test and design better methods of health service delivery, improve access to services, and provide continuity within the delivery system. Finally, they can assume leadership in training a new genre of health professionals whose functions are "synergistic" instead of competitive (Pellegrino, 1972, p. 4). The allied health occupations are well suited to these leadership roles because they are not as tradition bound as the older health occupations. Their relative youth and flexibility afford both educators and professional groups the chance to be in the forefront of change. Through their educational programs, they can help develop a health workforce that meets the service needs of the future effectively, efficiently, and humanely.

IV

Scope and Diversity of Allied Health Education

The provision of services for health care today requires an extraordinarily wide range of skills and knowledge. Allied health occupations differ with respect to the types of competencies required, ranging from the ability to perform routine tasks to comprehensive professional commitment to knowledge generation, and they also differ with respect to the scientific foundations of their knowledge base. Because of the numerous different types of allied health personnel who receive different didactic and clinical experiences in different settings, the present state of preparation for allied health occupations varies widely. Such variation in educational experiences occurs not only between health occupations but also, in some cases, for the same occupations. For some occupations, programs exist in a variety of educational settings, such as vocational-technical institutes, hospitals, and colleges. Sometimes academic units housing programs for the same occupations vary from one campus to another. Sometimes program length and/or award level may vary from one institution to another. Although one way is not necessarily correct and the other incorrect, the situation creates confusion for observers of allied health education in general and, more specifically, for educators, planners, and students.

To some extent, the confusion that exists today can be attributed to the rapid growth of allied health education in the 1960s, which often occurred with insufficient planning. Historical accounts by those who played a key role in the early development of allied health education tend to confirm the view that many programs were "developed at educational institutions [with] no previous experience in the health field, without access to adequate consultation, and lacking the potential for providing the required clinical learning experiences and other essential resources" (Kinsinger, 1973, p. 12). However, as the commission study progressed, it became increasingly apparent that much of the confusion is merely a reflection of the complexity of all that the term *allied health education* encompasses, and that the patterns that exist today are more rational than they seem.

This chapter takes a look at the growth and development of allied health education in the past, but the major focus is allied health education today and tomorrow. The essential components of allied health education are described, as well as the settings in which such education takes place. Special attention is given in the final section to schools and other administrative groupings of allied health programs in academic settings. These administrative units were explicitly designed to promote collaborative arrangements and to provide allied health students learning environments shared with others. Although they have not fulfilled all the highest expectations of the 1960s, these administrative units are built on valid premises and have achieved a great deal.

Growth and Change in Allied Health Education

An essential feature of allied health education since the 1960s has been rapid change and expansion, characterized by three major ingredients. First, there has been a tremendous proliferation of programs, particularly in collegiate settings, paralleling the huge expansion of two-year colleges and the growing popularity of vocational programs. In 1966, there were an estimated 2,500 collegiate programs; today there are over 8,000. Second, the distribution of programs has changed: Hospitals and other health service settings still play an active role, but the greatest growth in the number of programs has occurred in other settings, such as medical centers and universities, two-year colleges, vocational technical institutes, and private career schools. Third, the expansion of knowledge and skill requirements has led to greater diversification of education levels, now ranging from short-term certificate to full-fledged doctoral programs.

The patterns of education for allied health occupations have grown out of practice needs rather than resulting from an abstractly determined set of values. Thus the history of allied health education is closely related to the history of the occupations themselves. The rapid burgeoning of allied health occupations and education occurred in response to increasing national health service demands and the explosive growth in health science and technology. For example, the expansion of rehabilitation occupations grew in response to wartime needs and polio, and health physicists became established as an occupation with formal programs because hospitals needed such personnel to ensure safety and to meet accreditation standards. In such cases as radiologic technology and respiratory therapy, advances in technology required new types of personnel. Sometimes, as the scope of practice enlarged and it became practical or desirable to delegate tasks to others, a new cadre of health assistants and aides emerged.

No one pattern can describe the historical development of formal programs for allied health personnel; the influences have been varied and the forms of growth diverse. Perhaps the most frequently cited pattern is that associated with the early evolution of education for some occupations from employer-provided preceptorships to highly formalized collegiate-based programs. In the first phase, education consisted simply of learning to perform the tasks required by a particular employer, usually a physician's office or hospital. The training focused on application and was directly linked to service needs. Evaluation of learning was performance based and carried out by the practitioner, who functioned as a teacher, evaluator, role model, and employer.

The second phase began with the establishment of a professional association to represent the group identity and collective needs of the emerging occupational specialty and the formalization of education within the hospital. The heightening of occupational awareness typically led to sharp demarcation of boundaries, turf protection, tightening of entry requirements, initiation of credentialing processes, and movement away from apprenticeship-type settings. Moreover, the professionalization move was frequently marked by delegation of routine tasks to others, thus starting new occupations or a hierarchial differentiation of occupational levels.

The third stage began with increasing collaboration between hospitals and educational institutions, eventually culminating in a shift of programs to collegiate settings. This transition accelerated concerns about regulation, including accreditation of programs and certification of personnel. In addition to regulatory concerns, the needs and interests of the larger educational institutions exerted important influences. The shift to the collegiate setting brought a distinct demarcation of clinical and didactic education, which raised new issues, such as the value of theory versus practice, occupational preparation versus general education, and maintenance of flexibility in the face of constant innovation.

This pattern of growth is, of course, far from standard, even for occupations that were among the first to be recognized. Some allied health occupations still receive their preparation on the job; others are trained in hospital programs only. In many cases, these settings are the most appropriate, and further shifts are unlikely. Moreover, not all allied health programs were born in hospitals. Programs for some allied health personnel—such as those who work in the community to maintain and improve the general health through education, elimination or control of environmental hazards, management of health systems, and research and development—have emerged in nonhospital work settings or were conceived initially in collegiate settings.

The birth of occupational categories resulting from the establishment of new programs in collegiate settings is a relatively recent phenomenon and has been associated with an expanded knowledge base and/or expanded degree requirements. As admissions requirements change and students bring to collegiate programs competencies from prior coursework, the tendency is to raise the degree level and to create a new title. The new occupations at the higher level also spin off other occupations by delegating more routine tasks to others. New occupational levels sometimes evolve simultaneously with collegiate programs to fill new needs for advanced level practitioners, administrators, and teachers.

Formal programs for new occupations have also been developed by educators and other experts who believed that these occupations would help to meet special manpower needs. The preparation of physician assistants that began at Duke University in 1965 is a case in point. Today some institutions are experimenting with programs for generalists or persons with multiskills or cross-occupational competencies to reverse the splintering process which is seen as detrimental to effective health service delivery in many settings. One such generalist with a designated title is the circulation technologist; the occupation was conceived and delineated in academia. For the most part, the experimentation with multiskill or cross-occupational preparation has not, as yet, led to the spawning of new titles. However, new occupations are introduced and recognized regularly. For instance, in 1976 a unique pilot program to train spinal cord injury technicians was established in a Veterans Administration (VA) hospital to meet specific needs within the VA health care system (Administration of Veterans Affairs, 1977, p. 4). During 1978, the Committee on Allied Health Education and Accreditation (CAHEA) of the American Medical Association (AMA) initiated review procedures, recognizing anesthesiologist's assistants, cardiovascular perfusionists, and emergency medical technician-paramedics as emerging occupations (American Medical Association, 1978a, p. 1).

While new occupations are being introduced continuously, the more established ones are undergoing self-evaluation and organizational change. A project undertaken to delineate the roles and functions of respiratory therapy personnel from 1975 to 1978 found no substantial or consistent distinction between the practice characteristics of the certified respiratory technicians (graduates of approved training programs not less than one year in length) and registered respiratory therapists (graduates of approved training programs of two or more years). The project staff recommended a single, entry-level generalist position for certifying respiratory therapy practitioners (Jouette and others, 1978). The National Board for Respiratory Therapy studied this recommendation and endorsed the consolidation of registry and certification exams in June 1979. A second vote of approval by the board was given at their November 1979 meeting. This decision will be consolidated after 1983 and will change the educational requirements for both entry-level generalists and upper-level specialists.

In summary, allied health education is neither static nor sharply defined, but is rather a dynamic process, constantly responding to new health needs. Because allied health education must remain responsive to health service needs, it will be necessary for administrators and educators to plan explicitly for ongoing change and innovation. Therefore, openness and flexibility are essential requirements for allied health education. Such an open, divergent, and evolving field makes it essential for its practitioners to develop the capacity for constant evaluation and self-scrutiny. A major challenge for allied health educators in the coming decade will be to examine and test thoroughly the premises upon which current educational practices are based, with the courage to undertake revisions when necessary. Most difficult, perhaps, will be the development of the capacity to deal effectively with unanticipated changes—a problem apparently endemic to the health professions but one that is particularly acute within the allied health arena.

Components of Allied Health Education

A first objective of allied health education is to prepare students for an occupational role. A more difficult but equally important objective is to develop attitudes, as well as the capacity for lifelong learning. Allied health education cannot be confined to the acquisition of entry-level skills but must continue throughout one's career.

Basic occupational preparation programs prepare students for entry-level proficiency, following standards set by the educational programs. These entry-level skills generally require further refinement through on-the-job training or in-service programs at the place of work. In addition, the rapidly expanding knowledge base and developing technology make maintenance as well as improvement of competencies, through constant retooling and updating of skills, an essential component of the lifelong educational process. Specialization or acquisition of other skills may also become necessary for effective performance or career development. The commission endorses the concept of allied health education as a continuous rather than discrete process, with four components: (1) basic occupational preparation, (2) job education and training, (3) advanced education, and (4) continuing education. This scheme was derived from the work of the Task Force on Allied Health Clinical Education (1974) and policy statements of the American Hospital Association (1974).

Basic Occupational Preparation. Basic occupational preparation programs are designed to provide students with knowledge and skills needed to work in a specific occupation at the entry level of that occupation. Admission to the program does not require previous formal preparation in the occupation but may build on previous informal training or practical experience. Typically, this type of program grants the "first professional" degree which leads to a certificate or license, or prepares the student for an entry-level job. The program may be housed within a collegiate institution or given at a variety of other settings.

Basic occupational preparation programs vary depending on the types and ranges of practice skills needed but usually include a general education component, as well as both didactic and clinical preparation in an occupational area. The intensity and extent of the general education component varies in different occupations; in a collegiate program, it could include academic coursework in subjects such as English, mathematics, philosophy, language, fine arts, chemistry, biology, physics, and anatomy. For some occupations, such courses are electives; for others, they are essential as a knowledge base upon which to build occupational competencies. In shorter programs, the general education component may consist of health-related subject matters primarily (for example, medical terminology, basic health principles), which are not occupation specific but generic to all health professions. How much of general education is an essential component of allied health education leading to high quality practice is still a matter of subjective judgment.

The occupationally specific component includes studies and practice leading to the competencies required for entering the occupation. Occupational preparation generally includes a didactic component, which is mostly knowledge based and is taught in conventional educational environments, and a clinical one, which is practice based and is generally taught in actual work settings. Some aspects of clinical education can also be simulated and taught in the classroom or the laboratory. The integration of didactic and clinical components of allied health education remains a major concern; unresolved issues relating to control, quality, accessibility, and cost of clinical education are discussed in more detail in Chapter Six.

Basic occupational preparation programs are the major responsibility of educational institutions. However, health care agencies and other employers, as well as the armed forces, also provide such programs.

Job Education and Training. The objective of the basic occupational preparation program is to provide the student with the entry-level competencies needed for employment. The learning experiences will not and should not end with employment, however. All personnel will require some orientation, in-service education, and on-the-job training to function effectively within the employment setting.

The commission's survey of academic and clinical leaders found that on-the-job training was generally rated as more effective than formal education as preparation for a number of current activities. Although the basic occupational preparation programs provide a graduate with entry-level competencies and, in certain cases, broadly based skills, special on-the-job education or training programs are generally required to meet employer needs and to fit the graduate into the framework of the particular employer's procedures, systems, equipment, and facilities. In many health care institutions, staff in-service education includes a great deal more than just initial orientation to the job and the institution. Organized, ongoing programs provide continuing education at an advanced professional level. This pattern is not unique to health care personnel; it is true for occupational preparation programs in areas such as accounting and engineering as well (Bisconti and Solmon, 1976).

Job-specific preparation is the responsibility of employment settings, although in some instances employers have entered into cooperative arrangements with educational institutions to conduct these programs. These in-service programs should not be confused with clinical education, which also occurs in work settings. Clinical education is an integral part of the basic occupational preparation phase of the educational process and is distinct from job education or training programs.

Advanced Education. Advanced education for allied health personnel provides practitioners with formal education beyond that which is offered for basic occupational preparation. It may lead to additional clinical mastery and specialization or acquisition of nonclinical skills, such as teaching, administration, or research. Such education currently may be acquired in an allied health discipline or other areas, such as arts and sciences, education, or business. Thus the term *advanced education* is not limited to allied health programs but refers to formal postprofessional studies that supplement the basic occupational competencies of health personnel.

The importance of advanced education in the learning continuum should not be underrated. As the knowledge base for health occupations grows, there is a natural tendency to expand the entry-level requirements. A complete preparation in all aspects of a health discipline may not be necessary for entry-level work. Competencies learned but not used would not only be unnecessarily costly and wasteful but might also contribute to a feeling on the part of large numbers of practitioners that they are being underemployed. National data on college graduates in allied health and other fields show that one of the most important predictors of job satisfaction is a feeling that one's skills are fully utilized on the job (Bisconti and Solmon, 1977; Ochsner and Solmon, 1979).

For both cost considerations and fairness to students, it is appropriate to address basic occupational preparation to entry-level knowledge and skills and reserve for advanced education the knowledge and skills that are required only of the minority who perform advanced-level functions. Thus advanced education serves partly to build leadership capabilities by preparing teachers, administrators, and advanced clinicians and partly as a fundamental alternative to continual expansion of basic occupational preparation requirements.

Continuing Education. Continuing education for health professions is defined as any organized educational program or experience designed to assist a health care provider in maintaining or improving the level of competence necessary to perform current responsibilities in a manner consistent with the most recent advances in the field. Continuing education takes place after basic preparation for the occupation has been completed and thus overlaps, to some degree, with both advanced education and job training programs. As the number of continuing education courses designed to teach advanced competencies in clinical practice, management, and research has increased, the only real distinction between continuing and advanced education seems to have become whether the program awards continuing education units or academic degree credits. Moreover, many in-service education programs offered at health care institutions are formal continuing education programs.

Noncredit continuing education is the fastest growing segment of postsecondary education since the close of World War II. In 1975-76, according to estimates of the National Center for Education Statistics, there were over 700,000 registrations in academic health professions subjects offered as continuing education programs. Continuing education programs in "health services and paramedical technologies" enrolled over 280,000 students (Chronicle of Higher Education, 1978b, p. 1975). The same year, allied health programs in colleges and universities enrolled about 400,000 students and graduated about 100,000.

Unresolved problems and issues in continuing education include improved methods of assessing the relevance of course offerings to increased competence, control and evaluation of the process of continuing education, standardization of credit units, increased access, and the question of who is to pay if continuing education is mandatory. The public in general has high stakes in assuring continuing competency of health care personnel; this concern is reflected in increasing efforts to regulate such activities through recertification processes and mandatory continuing education. At the present time, for occupations in which continuing education is voluntary, the individual practitioner bears the responsibility to maintain clinical currency.

Continuing education programs are generally offered by academic institutions, professional associations, employers, and commercial groups. Because the purposes of continuing education are so obviously linked to practice, the growing recognition of continuing education has given impetus to competency-based approaches for allied health education in general. For instance, a major feature of the continuing education process is assessment of learning needs, so that the content is addressed to gaps in knowledge and skills. The individualized approach, based on the principle that students should be taught what they do not already know, has broad applicability for all four learning components. An increasing number of professional associations are also getting involved in testing and developing methods of self-assessment. An alternative to mandatory continuing education may be a requirement for periodic reassessment of competencies through examination.

In its broadest sense, then, the concept of allied health education denotes a continuous process—including four major components—the responsibility for which is shared by educational institutions, employers, professional associations, and the individual. This broader reality contrasts sharply with the narrower and more conventional understanding of allied health education as a set of programs housed in formal academic settings. The commission sought information on all four components of allied health education. Adequate information was available only for basic occupational preparation programs. Some data are available for advanced education programs designed specifically for allied health personnel, but there is no information on the extent of participation of allied health personnel in advanced education in other disciplines. Almost no data exist on the numbers and characteristics of job training and educational programs or continuing education programs. Despite the absence of data, however, there is a prevailing belief that the former are widespread and the latter are growing in number.

For the purposes of this study, allied health education was defined as any formal, postsecondary program in basic occupational preparation or advanced education for occupations listed in the ASAHP *Glossary* (see Appendix B). The following discussion includes information on the education for some nursing-related occupations, as well as special education services, because these categories were included in the *Glossary* and in the data base used to describe programs in collegiate settings. In addition, data from the American Hospital Association cover several occupations that are not included in the ASAHP *Glossary*.

Current Educational Scene

The formal postsecondary programs preparing allied health personnel are housed in a variety of settings. However, present efforts to describe these settings suffer from a lack of reliable data as severely as similar efforts of ten years ago. This is particularly true if one attempts to discuss changes over time and demonstrate the extent to which movement from one setting to another has occurred.

The commission worked with four major data sources on allied health education. ASAHP surveys of collegiate programs in 1973 and 1975, funded by the Bureau of Health Manpower, provide the most reliable national data on programs housed in the nation's colleges and universities. The American Hospital Association (AHA) surveys of hospital programs in 1973 and 1975, also funded by the Bureau of Health Manpower, provide comparable data on programs in hospital settings, but no data are available for programs in other health care institutions. The U.S. Office of Education (USOE) surveys in 1975 and 1977 of all postsecondary health occupational programs at the associate degree or lower-division certificate level provide information on programs housed in postsecondary noncollegiate institutions. Finally, the armed forces have data on the numbers and characteristics of allied health programs in the military.

Each data source, however, presented some problems, alone or when used for comparative purposes. For instance, some duplication in the counts of collegiate and hospital programs exists, probably inflating the number of programs in both settings. Further, no accurate information is available at present for collegiate or hospital programs prior to 1973. American Medical Association (AMA) records go back to the early 1960s but they include only accredited programs for a number of allied health occupations. Finally, ASAHP and AHA counts are based on survey responses, and population estimates can be made only with an appreciable margin of error.

The USOE data are not very comparable to ASAHP and AHA data, in that different titles for programs were used. Moreover, the USOE data underestimate the number of programs in noncollegiate settings because, when several programs were offered at an institution in an occupational area such as "medical/biological lab field," they were counted as one.

The armed forces provide probably the most accurate information of all; however, very little is known about the rate of transfer from the military to the civilian labor force. Finally, practically no information exists on other postsecondary programs conducted by various agencies with state or federal funds to train allied health personnel. There are about 800 allied health programs provided by various sponsors under the Comprehensive Employment and Training Act (CETA) (Kirschner Associates, 1977). This study of CETA-funded programs provides some information, but it is not clear to what extent the programs are at the postsecondary level.

Mase (1972) suggested that, when studying allied health, it would be better to go with "guesstimates" than with statistics that had no validity. What the commission has to offer is partially based on "guesstimates" and partially on statistics whose reliability is still questionable. In 1976, the latest year for which comparable survey information exists, there were about 14,000 formal postsecondary programs preparing allied health personnel. This figure is based on nearly 11,000 programs identified through the various surveys mentioned earlier and 3,000 estimated from survey nonresponse rates. Based on survey results and these estimates, 52 to 54 percent of allied health programs were housed in collegiate settings, 33 to 35 percent in hospitals, 10 to 12 percent in postsecondary noncollegiate institutions (for example, public vocational-technical institutes, private career schools), and one percent in the armed forces. Thus, by 1976, the collegiate settings had become the sector with the largest number of allied health programs.

Information provided to the commission by the American Medical Association demonstrates the gains in the collegiate sector. During the period from 1973 to 1977, the hospital sponsorship of AMA-accredited programs in twenty-three allied health occupations declined by 17 percent, from 1,940 to 1,614; in contrast, the number of AMA-accredited allied health programs sponsored by two-year colleges increased by 114 percent, from 276 to 590, and the number of four-year college programs by 39 percent, from 235 to 326.

It would be misleading to interpret this trend, as some have, as a change in the hospital's role in the education of allied health manpower. Undeniably there have been some shifts in training sites from hospitals to colleges and universities. Some of these shifts are due to the fact that a growing number of hospitals are now part of an academic health center, and they have become one component of a larger collegiate institution. Second, despite the shifts to collegiate settings, the number of hospital-based programs in some occupations has definitely grown. In fact, the absolute number of both hospital and collegiate programs has increased during the last decade, but the rate of increase has been much greater for collegiate programs than for hospital programs. For instance, during the period

1973 to 1976, the number of allied health programs in hospitals increased by 5 percent (Richter and Kosak, 1975; Kralovec, Williams, and Wilson, 1977) while the number of collegiate programs increased by 11 percent (Anderson and others, 1978). Moreover, hospital program directors surveyed in 1976 expected a slight decline in the number of graduates from their programs between 1976 and 1978, whereas collegiate program directors expected an increase. In 1976, the output of hospital programs was about 60 percent as great as that of collegiate programs; in 1978, this figure was expected to drop to just about 50 percent. Although hospital programs may now account for a smaller portion of all allied health programs than they did before, hospitals have not gotten out of the business of allied health education and are not likely to do so in the near future. Policy statements for AHA and the best available data clearly indicate that hospital training programs will continue to be important manpower sources, particularly for certain occupations, and that program offerings will fluctuate in accordance with employer needs.

Allied Health Programs in Colleges and Universities

In 1976, approximately 7,000 allied health programs were identified in the nation's institutions of higher education that met the following criteria: (1) award of a degree or certificate given as recognition of achievement, (2) students currently enrolled, and (3) at least thirty-six hours required for completion. An estimated 1,500 additional programs did not meet these criteria. The following account is based on 5,584 programs that responded to the ASAHP survey. About one fifth of the survey universe did not respond; thus this report excludes a substantial portion of formal ongoing collegiate programs. (See Appendix A for a discussion of methodology.)

Over half of the 3,000 higher education institutions in the United States had at least one allied health program (see Table 3). Public collegiate institutions were much more likely than private collegiate institutions to have allied health programs (71 percent of the former versus 37 percent of the latter

Table 3. Number and Percentage of Collegiate Institutions with Allied Health Programs in 1975-76, by Control and Type of Institution

	Higher Education Institutions[a]	With Allied Health Programs[b]	
		Number	Percent
Four-year colleges and universities—Total	*1,914*	*939*	*49*
Public	553	417	75
Private	1,361	522	38
Two-year colleges—Total	*1,141*	*684*	*60*
Public	901	609	68
Private	240	75	31
All collegiate institutions—Total	*3,055*	*1,623*	*53*
Public	1,454	1,026	71
Private	1,601	597	37

Sources: [a]*A Fact Book on Higher Education, Third Issue, 1976* (Washington, D.C.: American Council on Education, 1976).

[b]ASAHP 1976 Collegiate Inventory.

had at least one program). Two-year colleges, which had become an important educational site by 1975-76, were more likely than four-year collegiate institutions to have an allied health program (60 percent versus 49 percent respectively). Two-year colleges had 2,059 programs, and four-year colleges had 3,525 programs. Thus even though the number of four-year institutions in this country greatly outstrips the number of two-year institutions, nearly two in five collegiate allied health programs were in two-year colleges.

To determine more precisely which types of higher education institutions housed allied health programs, a 1976 version of the classification of higher education institutions developed by the Carnegie Commission on Higher Education (1973) was utilized. This classification identifies five relatively homogeneous categories of higher education institutions and a number of subcategories based upon their functions, as well as characteristics of their students and faculty. (See Appendix C for a description of this classification scheme.) Table 4 presents relevant information on the characteristics of allied health programs in higher education institutions based on the Carnegie Classification.

Table 4. Percent of Collegiate Institutions with Allied Health Programs in 1975-76, by Carnegie Classification of Institutional Type

Type of Institution	*Total Number of Such Institutions in the U.S.*	*Number and Percent with Allied Health Programs*		*Allied Health Programs*		*Mean Number of FTE Students per Institution*	*Mean Number Graduates per Institutions in 1975*	*Percent Offering Allied Health Programs*		*Percent Starting New Programs Between 1974-1976*
		Number	*Percent*	*Number*	*Mean Number per Institution*			*Prior to 1940*	*Prior to 1966*	
Research Universities I Leading universities in terms of federal financial support for academic science and award at least 50 Ph.D.s annually (and M.D.s if medical school on the same campus).	51	47	92	427	9	511	147	61	91	36
Research Universities II Among the leading 100 institutions in terms of federal financial support and award at least 50 Ph.D.s (and M.D.s if applicable).	47	41	87	288	7	319	91	36	87	18
Doctoral-Granting Universities I Award 40 or more Ph.D.s (and M.D.s) or received at least $3 million in total federal support in either 1969-70 or 1970-71. No institutions are included that grant fewer than 50 Ph.D.s (or M.D.s).	56	47	84	328	7	245	113	37	89	42
Doctoral-Granting Universities II Institutions awarding at least 10 Ph.D.s.	30	27	90	146	5	364	104	33	79	29

Comprehensive Universities and Colleges I Institutions offering a liberal arts program and several others (e.g., engineering, business administration); that have at least two professional or occupational programs, and enroll at least 2,000 students. Many have master's programs and, at most, limited doctoral programs.	380	302	79	1,222	4	149	52	9	58	31
Comprehensive Universities and Colleges II State colleges and some private colleges that offer a liberal arts program and at least one professional or occupational program such as nursing or teacher training, mainly with a degree in education.	217	135	63	282	2	43	12	4	47	23
Liberal Arts Colleges I Highly selective or among the 200 leading baccalaureate-granting institutions in terms of numbers of graduates receiving Ph.D.s at 40 leading doctoral-granting institutions.	126	27	21	40	2	50	9	18	64	14
Liberal Arts Colleges II Other liberal arts colleges, many of which are extensively involved in teacher training, granting degrees in arts and sciences rather than in education.	474	243	51	447	2	30	8	13	54	18

(continued on next page)

Table 4 (Continued)

Type of Institution	Total Number of Such Institutions in the U.S.	Number and Percent with Allied Health Programs		Allied Health Programs		Mean Number of FTE Students per Institution	Mean Number Graduates per Institutions in 1975	Percent Offering Allied Health Programs		Percent Starting New Programs Between 1974-1976
		Number	Percent	Number	Mean Number per Institution			Prior to 1940	Prior to 1966	
Two-Year Colleges and Institutions	1,135	671	59	1,889	3	65	53	1	21	35
Theological Seminaries, Bible Colleges, and Other Institutions Offering Degrees in Religion	277	5	2	4	1	47	57	0	50	25
Medical Schools and Medical Centers Includes only those that are listed as separate campuses in USOE *Opening Fall Enrollment*	51	35	69	212	6	415	110	39	76	58
Other Separate Health Professional Schools	29	7	24	9	1	60	23	0	31	17
Schools of Engineering and Technology Technical institutions are included only if they award a bachelor's degree and if their program is limited exclusively or almost exclusively to technical fields of study.	47	10	21	27	3	53	19	0	14	43

Schools of Business Management Included only if they award a bachelor's or higher degree and if their program is limited exclusively or almost exclusively to a business curriculum.	35	13	37	16	1	14	6	0	37	13
Schools of Art, Music, Design	58	2	3	3	2	33	6	0	0	0
Schools of Law	16	2	—	3	—	—	—	—	—	—
Teachers Colleges	28	5	18	17	3	135	87	20	60	20
Other Specialized Institutions Includes graduate centers, maritime academies, military institutions (lacking a liberal arts program), and miscellaneous.	35	3	9	9	3	29	26	50	50	0

Note: Updated version for 1975-76 based on Carnegie Commission on Higher Education (1973).

About half the programs were in university settings: 13 percent in highly prestigious Research University I and II categories (that contain most of the academic health centers), 9 percent in Doctoral-Granting Universities, and 23 percent in Comprehensive Universities and Colleges (a category that includes many state colleges with health professional training and teacher training programs). Highly selective Liberal Arts Colleges I had very few allied health programs but less selective Liberal Arts Colleges II had 8 percent of the programs. Two-year colleges shared about 35 percent of the programs, while single-campus medical schools had about 4 percent of the programs. (Multicampus medical schools are included in research university categories.)

Research and doctoral-granting universities as well as single-campus medical schools were likely to have a larger concentration of programs than were other types of schools. For instance, on the average, institutions in Research Universities I category had 9 programs in contrast to two-year colleges which had an average of only 3. At the program level, four-year colleges and universities tended to have smaller entering and graduating classes in allied health programs than did two-year colleges. However, at the institutional level, because of the concentration of programs, four-year colleges and universities had more students and graduates than did two-year colleges. An institution in the Research Universities I category had, on the average, 511 full-time-equivalent (FTE) students and 147 graduates. Single-campus medical schools had, on the average, 415 students and 110 graduates. In contrast, an average two-year college had 65 FTE students and 53 graduates. There appeared to be a greater concentration of allied health programs, students, and graduates in research and doctoral-granting universities as well as in single-campus medical schools than in other types of four-year institutions or two-year colleges. In fact, it is in these settings that the independent schools of allied health or other administrative allied health units, which will be discussed later in this chapter, are most likely to be housed.

Growth of Collegiate Programs. In 1976, just over six in ten allied health programs were in four-year colleges and universities, in contrast to over nine in ten in the 1950s. The participation of two-year colleges in allied health education is a relatively recent phenomenon. A comparison of program establishment dates reported in 1973-74 and 1975-76 ASAHP survey questionnaires shows that fully three in five allied health programs in four-year colleges and universities were established *before* 1970, whereas over three in five allied health programs in two-year colleges were established *after* 1970. The explosive growth of two-year colleges during the 1960s and early 1970s cannot fully account for the rapid increase of programs in two-year colleges. For instance, between 1974 and 1976, the increase in two-year colleges with allied health programs was much greater than the increase in two-year colleges in the nation as a whole, whereas the number of four-year colleges and universities with allied health programs did not keep pace with the overall growth of institutions of this kind.

The pioneering role of medical schools in establishing the early programs for allied health occupations is apparent. Over three fifths of Research Universities I, many of which have medical schools and teaching hospitals, started one or more allied health programs prior to 1940 (see Table 4). It is reasonable to assume that these programs were initiated at the teaching hospitals and then gradually moved to the medical school. Most of the research and doctoral-granting universities and single-campus medical schools that have some allied health programs today established at least one of these programs before 1966. The newcomers to the field of allied health education were two-year colleges, schools of engineering and technology, other health professional schools, and schools of business and management.

However, new programs were being added at all settings. Nearly three in five single-campus medical schools had started at least one new program between 1974 and 1976, as had two fifths of the Schools of Engineering and Technology and Doctoral-Granting Universities I. Over one third of Research Universities I and two-year colleges also had new programs. Despite these recent activities, the rapid growth of collegiate allied health programs that occurred during the period from 1965 to 1975 appears to have abated somewhat.

Occupational Categories. The 1975-76 ASAHP survey identified collegiate programs for 139 single occupational categories, grouped into 28 major areas. Of the 28 major occupational categories, 9 accounted for two thirds of the allied health programs in collegiate settings (see Table 5):

- clinical laboratory services, 17 percent
- administration, planning, and office, 8 percent
- health-related teacher preparation, 7 percent
- dental services, 7 percent
- speech and hearing services, 6 percent
- dietetic and nutritional services, 6 percent
- nursing-related services, 5 percent
- radiological services, 5 percent
- health education, 4 percent

About one in ten of the collegiate programs prepared medical technologists, the single occupation which had by far the largest number of programs (625). Radiologic technologist/technician and medical laboratory technician also accounted for a large number of collegiate programs. Nearly half the 139 occupational categories with programs in collegiate settings had fewer than 10 programs. Occupational categories with fewer than 10 programs tended to concentrate in such areas as information and communication, medical instrumentation and machine operation, pharmacy services, and vision care.

Out of 139 occupational categories, 45 percent had programs exclusively on four-year campuses and 12 percent on two-year campuses. The programs for the remaining 62 occupations were housed on the campuses of both four-year and two-year institutions. Finally, over two fifths of the programs in four-year colleges and three fifths of the programs in two-year colleges were not accredited. The difference in accreditation rates largely results from the concentration in two-year colleges of programs that had no accrediting bodies.

Types of Programs. A majority of the allied health programs responding to the ASAHP survey in 1975-76 were basic

Table 5. Allied Health Programs in Collegiate Institutions by Major Occupational Category: 1975-1976

Occupation Category	Total		Four-Year Colleges and Universities		Two-Year Colleges	
	Number	Percent	Number	Percent	Number	Percent
Administration, planning, and office	471	8	161	5	310	15
Biomedical engineering	97	2	76	2	21	1
Clinical laboratory services	931	17	739	21	192	9
Dental services	406	7	114	3	292	14
Dietetic and nutritional services	333	6	270	8	63	3
Emergency services	181	3	22	1	159	8
Environmental services	197	4	160	5	37	2
Health education	235	4	233	7	2	0+
Health-related teacher preparation	414	7	411	12	3	0+
Information and communication	30	1	30	1	0	0
Medical instrumentation and machine operation (other than respiratory therapy)	21	0+	9	0+	12	1
Medical record	155	3	65	2	90	4
Mental health	170	3	43	1	127	6
Nuclear medicine	49	1	39	1	10	1
Nursing-related services	294	5	52	2	242	12
Pharmacy services	5	0+	0	0	5	0+
Physician extender	61	1	48	1	13	1
Podiatric services	2	0	1	0	1	0
Radiological services	291	5	124	4	167	8
Rehabilitation—occupational	98	2	70	2	28	1
Rehabilitation—physical	186	3	144	4	42	2
Rehabilitation—other	100	2	83	2	17	1
Respiratory therapy services	194	4	62	2	132	6
Social services and counseling	151	3	113	3	38	2
Speech and hearing services	339	6	337	10	2	0+
Veterinary services	18	0+	3	0+	15	1
Vision care	51	1	16	1	35	2
Health professional—other	104	2	100	3	4	0+
Total	5,584	100	3,525	100+	2,059	100

Source: ASAHP 1976 Collegiate Inventory.

occupational preparation programs (85 percent); just one in ten were advanced education programs, 3 percent were teacher training programs, and fewer than one percent were continuing education programs (see Table 6). Advanced education and

Table 6. Distribution of Allied Health Programs in Four-Year and Two-Year Collegiate Institutions by Program Type: 1975-1976

	Total		*Four-Year Colleges and Universities*		*Two-Year Colleges*	
	Number	*Percent*	*Number*	*Percent*	*Number*	*Percent*
Basic occupational preparation	4,774	85	2,729	77	2,045	99
Advanced education	657	12	649	18	8	0+
Continuing education	12	0+	6	0+	6	0+
Teacher training	141	3	141	4		
Total	5,584	100	3,525	100	2,059	100

Source: ASAHP 1976 Collegiate Inventory.

teacher training programs generally were housed in four-year colleges and universities. Over half the programs in four-year colleges and universities awarded the baccalaureate degree, 23 percent the master's degree, and 5 percent the doctorate. However, 9 percent of the four-year college programs also awarded the associate degree and another 8 percent a certificate or diploma. In contrast, over three in five programs in two-year colleges awarded the associate degree and two in five the certificate or diploma (see Table 7).

Campus Settings for Programs. Although allied health programs were dispersed on a variety of campuses, there was clearly some relationship between the strengths of each campus setting and the type of occupational program. For instance, doctoral-granting institutions, with their strong arts and sciences schools, as well as medical schools and affiliated research hospitals, were more likely to have programs in clinical laboratory services, dental services, nutrition, environmental services, medical instrumentation and machine operations, and radiologic

Table 7. Award Levels of Allied Health Education Programs in Collegiate Institutions: 1975-1976

	Total		*Four-Year Colleges and Universities*		*Two-Year Colleges*	
Award Level	*Number*	*Percent*	*Number*	*Percent*	*Number*	*Percent*
Doctorate	182	3	182	5	–	–
Master's degree	799	14	799	23	–	–
Bachelor's degree	1,946	35	1,946	55	–	–
Associate degree	1,561	28	302	9	1,259	61
Certificate or diploma without degree	1,096	20	296	8	800	39
Total	5,584	100	3,525	100	2,059	100

Source: ASAHP 1976 Collegiate Inventory.

services. Programs for such research-oriented occupations as biostatistician, epidemiologist, toxicologist, and public health laboratory scientist also concentrated in doctoral-granting institutions, particularly in research university campuses. Finally, most of the programs for medical librarians and medical library assistants were also on the campuses of doctoral-granting institutions where most of the larger medical library facilities were located.

Comprehensive universities and colleges, which house most of the old teachers colleges, were the setting for a majority of the programs in health education and health-related teacher preparation. They also contained a majority of the programs in vision care services, speech and hearing services, respiratory therapy, and some of the programs in mental health, medical records, and information and communication. In general, at comprehensive universities and colleges, more programs were at the technician level than at the technologist level; at doctoral-granting institutions, the opposite was true.

Liberal arts colleges, with their excellent biological science departments, housed most of the programs in medical technology and microbiology technology. Their social science departments housed most of the programs for mental health associates, art and dance therapists, and psychiatric social workers. These colleges also had a majority of the programs for the dietetic assistant (included in the home economics program) and the medical transcriptionist (as part of the secretarial program).

The academic units in which allied health programs were located ranged from medical schools to schools of arts and sciences. About half the allied health programs were housed in some organizational unit clearly identified as health (see Table 8). Just under one fifth of the programs were housed in a unit

Table 8. Distribution of Collegiate Programs Within Various Organizational Units

Organizational Unit	*Number*	*Percent*
Health-Related—Total	*2,037*	*54*
Allied or associated health[a]	669	18
Medical school/not in allied health unit	158	4
Dentistry	56	1
Other health unit	1,154	31
Other—Total	*1,744*	*46*
Arts and sciences	880	23
Education	431	11
Vocational studies	171	5
Engineering	96	3
Home economics	62	2
Agriculture	29	1
Secretarial	8	0+
Other	67	2
Total	3,781[b]	100

[a]Only those academic units with "allied health" or "associated health" included in their titles.

[b]Includes only programs for which organizational location was given.

Source: ASAHP 1976 Collegiate Inventory.

(college, school, or division) with "allied health" or "associated health" in its title. This figure can be considered small or large depending on one's perspective. Given the fact that the allied health education concept was barely ten years old in 1976, the concentration of even one fifth of the programs under an allied health umbrella is remarkable. Such units contained about half the programs in pharmacy services, physician assistant services, and vision care, as well as about two fifths of the programs in medical instrumentation and machine operation, nuclear medicine, radiologic services, and occupational and physical therapy. Only a small proportion of medical technology programs were in allied health units, but because of the large number of such programs overall, they represented nearly one fifth of all programs in such units.

Collegiate Output. Total enrollments in the collegiate allied health programs identified by the 1975-76 ASAHP survey were 280,531. The mean number of students per program was about 50, but half the programs had 20 or fewer students. Adjusting for the fact that about 1,500 programs did not respond to the ASAHP survey could add another 40,000 to 80,000 students to the 280,531 figure, bringing the total to just under 400,000. Thus, in 1976, the students in allied health programs comprised about 2 to 4 percent of 11 million degree-credit and nondegree-credit enrollments in colleges and universities.

Women predominated among students enrolled in allied health programs; they composed about three fourths of the students in both two-year and four-year institutions. Occupational areas with the highest proportions of women were medical records, rehabilitation (occupational), dental services, dietetic and nutritional services, nursing-related services, and veterinary services. Women were the minority, however, in biomedical engineering, environmental services, emergency services, vision care, and physician assistant services.

One out of every ten students enrolled in basic occupational programs in 1976 was black, but there was wide variation in the proportions of blacks enrolled in different program levels and curriculum areas. Black students composed only 8 percent of enrollments in basic occupational allied health programs in four-year colleges and universities, compared with 12 percent in two-year college programs. Consequently, they were substantially underrepresented in the pipeline for therapist or technologist-level allied health occupations and slightly overrepresented in the pipeline for those occupations requiring less training. Areas of study having relatively high proportions of black students include mental health, medical records, dietetic and nutritional services, respiratory therapy, health education, and nursing-related services. Those with particularly low proportions of black students were biomedical engineering, dental services, environmental services, physician assistant services, and rehabilitation (occupational). Black students were best represented in majors associated with a community health orientation or with employment in a hospital. In general, blacks tended to be poorly represented in programs preparing students for work in doctors' or dentists' offices. Part of the explanation may be the relatively poor representation of blacks among health professionals in private practice. In addition, after almost two decades of relatively intense minority recruitment efforts, blacks compose less than 7 percent of the total medical college enrollment (Office of Graduate Medical Education, 1979). The scarcity of role models at the top of the career structures in private practice and in the educational settings undoubtedly offers little encouragement to black students to prepare for related allied health careers. A similar case can be made for Hispanic Americans, as well as other disadvantaged ethnic groups.

Collegiate allied health programs responding to the survey graduated about 80,000 students in 1976. The total number of graduates from all of the programs in collegiate settings was probably in excess of 100,000. Although the collegiate sector accounted for over one half of the programs in allied health education, they might have contributed less than one half of the graduate output. Accreditation standards and other academic requirements constrain the number of students that participate in academic programs. This is in contrast to the allied health programs housed in private career schools, which concentrate on short-term programs offered more than once each year, or military programs which, although few in number (127), produce over 30,000 graduates annually.

Advanced Education Programs in Collegiate Settings. As mentioned earlier, advanced education for allied health personnel provides practitioners with formal education beyond that which is offered as basic occupational preparation. In general usage, the term *advanced education* refers to study beyond the baccalaureate; however, for allied health occupations, this is not necessarily the case. For example, for personnel prepared at the associate degree level, advanced preparation usually involves education leading to a bachelor's degree. Advanced education, then, denotes the sequential aspect of additional studies beyond the requirements of basic occupational preparation but does not specify the degree level. There are, however, some exceptions to this sequential pattern. Some overlap between basic occupational preparation programs and advanced education occurs when a basic occupational preparation program is geared also to competencies (such as administration or teaching) which are not required for entry level (for example, four-year dental hygiene programs combine entry-level preparation for clinical work and additional preparation for academic employment).

Kingston (1978) describes five major types of advanced education for allied health practitioners: (1) basic science degree programs in an area of science directly related to the technical basis of a particular profession; (2) advanced skills degree programs in a specialty area; (3) general education or administration degree programs; (4) allied health education and administration degree programs, and (5) two-plus-two programs in general education and administration for those with associate degrees or certificates (see Table 9). Only the second and possibly the fourth of these five types can be identified as advanced education programs in allied health disciplines, but all five are advanced educational experiences for allied health personnel, offering them opportunities for career growth and development.

Table 9. Types of Collegiate Programs in Advanced Education for Allied Health Personnel

Types of Programs	*Examples*	*Objectives*
1. Basic science degree programs in areas of science directly related to the technical basis of particular professions	Master's program in microbiology for medical technologists Master's program in physiology for physical therapists	To increase professional qualifications by giving the background in the sciences basic to the health care skills

(continued on next page)

Table 9 (Continued)

Types of Programs	*Examples*	*Objectives*
2. Programs offering an advanced skills degree in a specialty area	Master's program in orthopedics and pediatrics for physical therapists Graduate-degree programs in clinical skills related to children's dentistry or periodontics for dental hygienist	To prepare the student for clinical specialization To prepare the student for teaching or research
3. General education or administration degree programs	Training in such fields as business administration or education that does not necessarily enable allied health students to expand or refine their skills as practitioners	To prepare the student for administration or teaching
4. Education and administration program for allied health professionals	Training in such fields as business administration and education that is specifically designed for allied health professionals with a minor in advanced training in an allied health discipline	To prepare the student for teaching or administration
5. 2 + 2 programs	Education or administration programs for allied health practitioners who have only the two-year or associate degree Education or administration programs combined with a minor in advanced skills in a specific occupation	 To enable the student to advance in practice

Source: Kingston, 1978, p. 87.

The 1975-76 ASAHP survey provides some information on advanced education programs that were offered by the departments surveyed. ASAHP defined advanced education as any "program designed to provide health workers with formal education or training beyond that which is offered as 'Basic Occupational Preparation,' AND which confers additional academic credit or professional recognition in a specific discipline or occupation. This type of program includes Specialty Training which qualifies the individual in a recognized specialty of his discipline, for which there are specific educational requirements beyond 'Basic Occupational Preparation' " (Anderson, Nunn, and Sedlacek, 1976, p. 83). Out of a total of 5,584 allied health programs, 12 percent (or 649) were identified as advanced education programs by the program directors responding to the survey. These programs covered all major allied health occupational categories, with the exception of pharmacy services, podiatric services, and veterinary services. The vast majority of the advanced programs were at the graduate level; only 6 percent led to the baccalaureate, and 4 percent to an undergraduate certificate. Of the 596 graduate-degree level programs, 70 percent were at the master's level, 27 percent at the doctoral level, and about 3 percent were certificate programs for advanced standing (see Table 10).

The largest number of advanced education programs designed specifically for allied health personnel were in health-related teacher preparation (109 programs), dietetic and nutritional services (77 programs), environmental services (67 programs), and health education (52 programs). Three fourths were located in public four-year colleges and universities and almost all the others in private four-year institutions. Just one percent were in two-year colleges. The programs were spread in many different campus locations, with the highest concentration (29 percent) in health-related schools and divisions: 8 percent in an organizational unit with allied health in the title, 4 percent in a school of medicine, and most of the remainder in a school of public or community health. About 13 percent of the programs were in schools of education (mostly special educa-

Table 10. Advanced Education Programs in Collegiate Settings, by Program Award Level, 1975-1976

Award Level	Programs: Number	Programs: Percent
Certificate—Total	*15*	*2*
Certificate I (0-5 months)	1	0+
Certificate II (6-11 months)	3	1
Certificate III (12-23 months)	9	1
Certificate IV (24-36 months)	2	0+
Bachelor's Degree/Certificate—Total	*38*	*6*
Bachelor's degree	22	3
Bachelor's degree and certificate	2	0+
Collegiate certificate	14	2
Advanced Degree/Certificate—Total	*596*	*92*
Master's degree	391	60
Master's degree and certificate	27	4
Certificate of advanced standing	15	2
Doctoral degree	163	25
Total	649	100

Source: ASAHP Collegiate Inventory.

tion) and 10 percent in schools of engineering (mostly environmental engineering). Other locations given for these programs related to home economics, arts and humanities, social and behavioral sciences, applied sciences, agriculture, pharmacy, and library science. The location of nearly one third of the programs was not given or referred to merely as "graduate school."

About 23,000 students were enrolled in these advanced education programs, about two fifths on a part-time basis. Those in undergraduate certificate and baccalaureate programs were most likely to be enrolled full time. Nearly half the master's and graduate certificate students were enrolled part time; apparently many were employed while working toward their master's degree. However, doctoral studies seemed to demand heavier concentration, as only one fifth of the students in doctoral programs were enrolled part time. On the average, each advanced education program had an enrollment of 36: 22 full-time students and 14 part-time students.

Kingston (1978, p. 88) has argued that advanced education programs in allied health grew haphazardly over the last decade: "New graduate degrees have been offered through whatever department of college could arrange them and in whatever curriculum design was available. While this spurt of growth has been necessary, given the pressure for more qualified personnel in many areas of the health care delivery system, the lack of comprehensive planning has produced a variety of new advanced degree programs whose location and content must be described as irregular at best. (The quality of these programs is an additional issue.)" (Kingston, 1978, p. 88). The ASAHP survey results do not entirely support Kingston's assertion about a "spurt of growth": Of the 500 programs identified as advanced, 29 percent were established prior to 1960, 38 percent between 1960 and 1970, and only one third since 1970. More information is needed, however, to comment on the quality of these programs.

The commission survey of academic and clinical leaders showed that most of those who had achieved eminence in allied health education and practice held graduate degrees. All the academic leaders held such degrees; most held a doctorate. Since graduate degrees in allied health disciplines are relatively new, it is not surprising that almost all the degrees were in other disciplines; two fifths were health related (for example, psychology, public health, medicine) and most of the others were in educational administration or natural or biological sciences. Among the clinical leaders, about seven in ten held a graduate degree and 42 percent held a doctorate. Nearly three fifths of these degrees were health related, and the remainder were in business, education, and administration.

Most of the academic and clinical leaders agreed that the route to leadership positions in allied health included basic preparation in allied health or health-related fields, followed by work experience (clinical practice and/or teaching), which in turn was followed by formal training in administration or business management. Advanced education, whether in administration and education or in clinically related fields, was an essential part. One interesting finding of this survey was that women, who constitute the majority among students and practitioners in many allied health categories, were underrepresented among the leadership in the field. This can be partially explained by the fact that women are still underrepresented among those with advanced degrees in allied health. For instance, according to the National Center for Education Statistics (Chronicle of Higher Education, 1978a, p. 197), 67,612 persons earned a bachelor's or higher degree in 1976 in "health professions" (all health-related disciplines except medicine, dentistry, optometry, osteopathic medicine, podiatry, and veterinary medicine): 80 percent were bachelor's degrees, 19 percent master's degrees and just about one percent doctorates. Women constituted 79 percent of those earning the baccalaureate, 66 percent of those earning the master's, but only 29 percent of those earning the doctorate. Unless women are encouraged to pursue higher degrees, their representation among the leadership in allied health is bound to remain small. A similar case can be made for blacks and other ethnic minorities. Solid credentials are required for any group that has been excluded from leadership positions to assume a position of power and eminence.

Allied Health Programs in Hospital Settings

In a policy statement in 1974, the American Hospital Association explicitly stated that every hospital and other health care agency in the nation has a legal and moral obligation to ensure that those who provide services are competent. Included within this responsibility are the in-service programs, job training, and continuing education programs discussed earlier in this chapter. Although basic occupational preparation was seen primarily as the responsibility of educational institutions, the American Hospital Association (1974, p. 2) asserted that

> under certain circumstances, hospitals and other health care agencies must assume primary responsibility, including financing, for such preparatory education. Such circumstances can include any of the following elements:
> - A suitable educational institution does not exist in the area.

- Existing educational institutions are unable or unwilling to provide preparatory education programs.
- Existing educational institutions are unable to produce a sufficient number of graduates to meet manpower needs.
- Programs offered by hospitals and other health care agencies are better than other available programs in terms of generally accepted measures of cost to the community and of competence of graduates.

In 1976, over one third of the allied health programs were in hospitals. This count does not include clinical education programs, internships, or residencies. Next to providing health care, education appears to be the second major function of hospitals; further, it is a function which, contrary to some prevailing opinions, has been growing rather than diminishing—at least until 1976. A comparison of 1973 and 1976 surveys clearly indicates increases in educational activities, regardless of hospital size. In fact, the largest increase was reported by those with fewer than fifty beds; thus even smaller hospitals seem to be taking on an education function.

Educational programs in hospitals cover a wide scope of occupational areas and range from marginally formal to highly structured. Program scheduling reflects the needs of the hospital: Two fifths of the programs are conducted on a need basis; another two fifths are conducted once a year, and the remaining ones are conducted more than once a year or follow another schedule, depending on staff vacancies. Only one third of the programs are restricted to hospital employees (two thirds are open to all), and fully seven in ten are free, charging no tuition. Nine in ten programs require high school graduation as a prerequisite. A majority of the programs confer either a certificate of completion, diploma, associate degree, bachelor's degree, or master's degree; some confer multiple awards. Two fifths of the programs are accredited or in the process of accreditation review (Kralovec, Williams, and Wilson, 1977).

The 1976 AHA *Directory* reported about 3,800 programs that provided training in 82 health occupations corresponding to the categories in the ASAHP *Glossary*. Those occupations listed as nursing-related occupations (nurse aide, nurse practitioner, and the like) composed 27 percent of the programs—followed by clinical laboratory services (16 percent), radiologic services (13 percent), and administration, planning, and office work (12 percent) (see Table 11). On the average, hospital programs were nine months in length (see Table 12). However, there was considerable variation in program length both within single occupations and between occuptions. Programs over twelve months in length included those for radiologic services, vision care, dental services, physician assistants, speech and hearing, nuclear medicine, and clinical laboratory services.

Table 11. Allied Health Programs in Hospitals by Major Occupational Category: 1975-1976

	Number	*Percent*
All major occupational categories	*3,779*	*100*
Nursing and related services	1,020	27
Clinical laboratory services	617	16
Radiological services	494	13
Administration, planning, and office	449	12
Mental health	215	6
Dietetic and nutritional services	195	5
Social services and counseling	174	5
Medical instrumentation and machine operation	163	4
Respiratory therapy services	119	3
Emergency services	113	3
Nuclear medicine	78	2
Pharmacy services	67	2
Medical record	34	1
Rehabilitation (physical)	11	0+
Physician extender	7	0+
Rehabilitation (other)	6	0+
Vision care	5	0+
Information and communication	3	0+
Rehabilitation (occupational)	3	0+
Dental services	2	0
Speech and hearing services	2	0
Biomedical engineering	1	0
Veterinary services	1	0

Source: Kralovec, Williams, and Wilson, 1977.

Table 12. Hospital-Based Allied Health Programs: 1975-1976

Title of the Program	*Number*	*Length (Mos.)* *Range*	*Length (Mos.)* *Average*	*Percent Accredited*	*Total Enroll-ment*	*Average Number Students Per Program*	*1975 Graduates*	*Average Number Graduates Per Program*
Administration, Planning and Office	*440*		*2.1*	*0.0*	*734*	*1.7*	*5,319*	*12.1*
Hospital assist. administrator	2	12-18	15.0	0.0	5	2.5	4	2.0
Medical/dental secretary	1	12	12.0	0.0	3	3.0	0	0.0
Unit clerk	414	1-8	1.9	0.0	705	1.7	5,241	12.7
Unit manager	23	1-8	3.1	0.0	21	0.9	74	3.2
Biomedical Engineering	*1*		*6.0*	*0.0*	*0*	*0.0*	*0*	*0.0*
Biomedical engineering technician	1	6	6.0	0.0	0	0.0	0	0.0
Clinical Lab Services	*577*		*12.3*	*87.9*	*3,536*	*6.1*	*3,624*	*6.3*
Spec. in blood bank technology	19	12-18	12.6	89.5	49	2.6	46	2.4
Chemistry technologist	1	15	15.0	0.0	13	13.0	2	2.0
Cytotechnologist	50	6-13	11.9	100.0	193	3.9	200	4.0
Electron microscopy tech.	1	11	11.0	0.0	5	5.0	5	5.0
Hematology technologist	3	6-12	10.0	0.0	15	5.0	15	5.0
Histologic technician	65	6-36	12.4	76.9	111	1.7	110	1.7
Medical lab assistant	56	1-24	11.5	78.6	283	5.1	343	6.1
Medical lab technician	20	6-24	16.5	45.0	91	4.6	85	4.3
Medical technologist	361	12-14	12.2	93.4	2,775	7.7	2,818	7.8
Microbiology technologist	1	12	12.0	0.0	1	1.0	0	0.0
Dental Services	*2*		*16.5*	*50.0*	*7*	*3.5*	*5*	*2.5*
Dental assistant	1	9	9.0	100.0	5	0.5	5	5.0
Maxilloracial prosthodontic technician	1	24	24.0	0.0	2	0.2	0	0.0

(continued on next page)

Table 12 (Continued)

Title of the Program	Number	Length (Mos.) Range	Length (Mos.) Average	Percent Accredited	Total Enroll-ment	Average Number Students Per Program	1975 Graduates	Average Number Graduates Per Program
Dietetic and Nutritional Services	*182*		*10.1*	*72.5*	*752*	*4.1*	*1,387*	*7.6*
Dietary aide	33	1-12	3.9	0.0	144	4.4	691	20.9
Dietetic assistant	6	2-13	8.0	16.7	23	3.8	32	5.3
Dietetic technician	8	1-12	5.4	12.5	52	6.5	105	13.1
Dietitian	133	6-24[a]	12.0	96.2	515	3.9	535	4.0
Nutritionist	2	7-9	8.0	100.0	18	9.0	24	12.0
Emergency Services	*108*		*4.5*	*0.0*	*2,484*	*23.0*	*5,626*	*52.1*
Ambulance attendant	3	1-8	4.0	0.0	25	8.3	43	14.3
Emergency medical technician	105	1-15	4.5	0.0	2,459	23.4	5,583	52.2
Information and Communication	*3*		*16.0*	*0.0*	*8*	*2.7*	*4*	*1.3*
Medical photographer	3	16	16.0	0.0	8	2.7	4	1.3
Medical Instrumentation and Machine Operations	*157*		*6.5*	*3.8*	*211*	*1.3*	*424*	*2.7*
Cardiopulmonary technician	10	3-12	6.2	0.0	16	1.6	36	3.6
Circulation technologist	2	18-24	21.0	0.0	5	2.5	5	2.5
Dialysis technician	32	1-12	5.0	0.0	63	2.0	109	3.4
Electrocardiographic technician	59	1-12	4.2	0.0	67	1.1	183	3.1
Electroencephalographic/cardiographic technician	8	2-13	8.6	0.0	5	0.6	11	1.4
Electroencephalographic technologist/technician	44	1-36	9.9	13.6	55	1.3	78	1.8
Pulmonary function technician	2	1-6	3.5	0.0	0	0.0	2	1.0
Medical Record	*34*		*6.3*	*5.9*	*108*	*3.2*	*189*	*5.6*
Medical record administrator	1	11	11.0	100.0	16	16.0	16	16.0
Medical record technician	5	3-12	6.4	20.0	24	4.8	22	4.4
Medical transcriptionist	28	1-12	6.2	0.0	68	2.4	151	5.4

Mental Health	*198*		*4.5*	*0.0*	*1,461*	*7.4*	*7,347*	*37.1*
Human services technologist/technician	1	13	13.0	0.0	0	0.0	30	30.0
Mental health administrator	2[b]	4-6	5.0	0.0	0	0.0	2	1.0
Mental health assoc./technician/assistant	16	2-24	8.1	0.0	172	10.7	688	43.0
Mental health technologist	10[b]	2-12	5.2	0.0	17	1.7	411	41.1
Mental retardation aide	17	1-12	4.7	0.0	283	16.6	1,470	86.5
Psychiatric technician	152	1-22	4.0	0.0	989	6.5	4,746	31.2
Nuclear Medicine	*72*		*12.7*	*100.0*	*381*	*5.3*	*319*	*4.4*
Nuclear medical technologist/technician	72	12-24	12.7	100.0	381	5.3	319	4.4
Nursing Related Services	*955*		*5.1*	*14.1*	*3,691*	*3.9*	*19,120*	*20.0*
Geriatric care worker	2	1-2	1.5	0.0	0	0.0	7	3.5
Nurse aide/orderly	685[b]	1-12	2.1	0.0	2,055	3.0	17,808	26.0
Nurse anesthetist	106	18-25	22.6	100.0	1,080	10.2	608	5.7
Nurse midwife	1	8	8.0	100.0	13	13.0	16	1.6
Nurse practitioner	17	3-12	8.5	0.0	109	6.4	119	7.0
Obstetrical technician	15	1-6	3.1	0.0	22	1.5	20	1.3
Operating room technician	129	1-18	6.8	21.7	412	3.2	542	4.2
Vision Care	*5*		*20.6*	*80.0*	*16*	*3.2*	*14*	*2.8*
Ophthalmic asst./technician	2	7-24	15.5	50.0	7	3.5	9	4.5
Orthoptist	3	24	24.0	100.0	9	3.0	5	1.7
Pharmacy Services	*65*		*5.8*	*0.0*	*130*	*2.0*	*290*	*4.5*
Medication pharmacy technician	5	3-12	7.0	0.0	34	6.8	32	6.4
Pharmacy technician	60[b]	1-24	5.7	0.0	96	1.6	258	4.3
Physician Extender	*6*		*15.0*	*33.3*	*84*	*14.0*	*18*	*3.0*
Physician assistant—primary care	4	6-24	18.0	50.0	79	19.8	13	3.2
Physician assistant—specialty	2	6-12	9.0	0.0	5	2.5	5	2.5
Radiologic Services	*466*		*23.4*	*98.7*	*6,101*	*13.1*	*3,000*	*6.4*
Radiation therapy technologist/technician	28	12-24	14.1	100.0	75	2.7	53	1.9
Radiologic technologist/technician	435	12-30	24.0	99.3	6,023	13.8	2,947	6.8
Ultrasound technical specialist	3	12-24	16.0	0.0	3	1.0	0	0.0

(continued on next page)

Table 12 (Continued)

Title of the Program	Number	Length (Mos.) Range	Length (Mos.) Average	Percent Accredited	Total Enroll-ment	Average Number Students Per Program	1975 Graduates	Average Number Graduates Per Program
Rehabilitation—Occupational	*3*		*2.7*	*0.0*	*1*	*0.3*	*5*	*1.7*
Occupational therapist	2	3	3.0	0.0	1	0.5	4	2.0
Occupational therapy assistant	1	2	2.0	0.0	0	0.0	1	1.0
Rehabilitation—Physical	*11*		*14.7*	*0.0*	*26*	*2.4*	*66*	*6.0*
Orthopedic technician	2	7-12	9.5	0.0	2	1.0	10	5.0
Orthotic/prosthetic technician	2	24-27	25.5	0.0	2	1.0	0	0.0
Orthotist/prosthetist	2	24-48	36.0	0.0	7	3.5	0	0.0
Physical therapist	1	2	2.0	0.0	11	11.0	37	37.0
Physical therapy assistant	4	2-6	4.5	0.0	4	1.0	19	4.8
Rehabilitation—Other	*5*		*5.2*	*0.0*	*9*	*1.3*	*8*	*1.6*
Art therapist	1	9	9.0	0.0	3	3.0	3	3.0
Music therapist	1	6	6.0	0.0	4	4.0	2	2.0
Recreational therapist	3	2-6	3.7	0.0	2	0.7	3	1.0
Respiratory Therapy Services	*104*		*10.1*	*50.0*	*668*	*6.4*	*637*	*6.1*
Respiratory therapist	11	3-24	15.4	81.3	176	16.0	118	10.7
Respiratory therapy technician	93	1-24	9.5	46.2	492	5.3	519	5.6
Social Services and Counseling	*170*		*6.9*	*78.2*	*922*	*5.4*	*1,879*	*11.0*
Alcohol/drug abuse specialist	18	3-14	10.1	0.0	210	11.7	270	15.0
Child care worker	4	5-6	5.7	0.0	48	12.0	120	30.0
Clinical pastoral counselor	139	3-24	6.3	95.7	607	4.4	1,430	10.3
Family counselor	1	12	12.0	0.0	36	36.0	6	6.0
Homemaker/home health aide	3	1	1.0	0.0	0	0.0	31	10.3
Medical social worker	2	9-18	13.5	0.0	9	4.5	7	3.5
Psychiatric social worker	1	12	12.0	0.0	5	5.0	6	6.0
Rehabilitation counselor	1	12	12.0	0.0	4	4.0	6	6.0
Social work associate	1	24	24.0	0.0	3	3.0	2	2.0

Speech and Hearing Services	*2*		*15.0*	*0.0*	*2*	*1.0*	*2*	*1.0*
Audiologist	1	15	15.0	0.0	1	1.0	1	1.0
Speech pathologist	1	15	15.0	0.0	1	1.0	1	1.0
Veterinary Services	*1*		*4.0*	*100.0*	*15*	*15.0*	*18*	*18.0*
Laboratory animal worker	1	4	4.0	100.0	15	15.0	18	18.0
Total	3,567		9.0	42.2	21,347	6.0	49,301	13.8

Note: Clinical portions of some academic programs may be included, thus inflating the number of hospital programs. Enrollments refer to programs operating as of April 15, 1976, thus underestimate annual enrollment count. Table includes programs that responded to all questions; therefore, the total numbers of programs, students, and graduates are underestimated.

[a]Not specified.

[b]Multilevel programs.

Source: American Hospital Association, 1977a.

Programs under six months in length included pharmacy services, emergency services, mental health, and administration, planning and office work. Some programs, such as that for nurse aides, had marked variations in length. The mean number of graduates per program in hospital settings was 14 but varied from mental retardation aide programs, averaging 86, and emergency medical technician programs, averaging 52, to speech and hearing services and information and communication services, which averaged fewer than 2 graduates in each. Again the small numbers of graduates reflect the hospital policy to train only what they need.

As mentioned earlier, program directors expected a decrease in graduate output from 63,935 in 1976 to 60,039 in 1978. The major reductions were planned for programs for nurse aide and unit clerks, which had registered reductions since 1973. Programs for emergency medical technicians and psychiatric technicians were also headed for cutbacks. These reductions may signal long-term changes in manpower demand but they can also reflect short-term variations in hospital employment patterns. For instance, the number of graduates from radiologic technology programs was reduced by 14 percent during the period from 1973 to 1976; yet, in 1976, program directors were planning a 20 percent increase in the number of graduates by 1978. These changes should be viewed as an example of the flexibility of hospital programs to respond directly to varying manpower needs. Clearly, this is a major advantage of hospital programs—an advantage shared with postsecondary noncollegiate institutions but one that is not a characteristic of collegiate programs. Another advantage of hospital-based allied health programs lies in the opportunities afforded to disadvantaged students: Many hospital-based programs not only are tuition free but also provide free or subsidized housing, meals, uniforms, and, in some cases, a stipend. This has permitted many disadvantaged students to enter health fields such as respiratory therapy or radiologic technology when they could not have afforded collegiate tuition or lived without some subsidy. Collegiate programs have closed the doors into health service occupations for many disadvantaged students because of their increasingly stringent admissions requirements and costs.

Finally, as mentioned earlier, a number of hospitals are now part of an academic health center and have increasing contact with collegiate policies, philosophies, standards, and resources. In addition, many other hospital-based programs have arrangements with local collegiate institutions to permit students in the hospital programs to take some courses for college credit. These arrangements are most often made with two-year colleges and have obvious value in facilitating career mobility and letting hospital program students have some contact with a broader mixture of faculty, students, and subjects. Collaboration between hospitals and collegiate institutions has now become quite frequent and is likely to grow in response to increasing pressures toward cost-effectiveness and quality control.

Allied Health Programs in Postsecondary Noncollegiate Institutions

In 1976, over 10 percent of allied health programs were housed in postsecondary noncollegiate institutions—a group of 11,000 highly heterogeneous little-known institutions. Until 1972, higher education generally meant collegiate institutions. Almost all research on higher education concerned the fewer than 3,000 four-year and two-year colleges and universities and excluded all other postsecondary institutions. The 1972 Education Amendments made noncollegiate institutions eligible for public funds and forced the recognition of these institutions as an integral part of postsecondary education. Even today, *higher education* is most often used to refer specifically to traditional collegiate institutions, whereas *postsecondary* is a more generic term used to denote any formal study preceding completion of secondary education.

In 1973, the National Commission on the Financing of Postsecondary Education surveyed the noncollegiate sector and found that the great majority (9,000 out of 11,000) were profit-making or proprietary schools; the remainder were public vocational-technical institutes and trade schools (Youn and Thompson, 1974). There are major differences between private proprietary schools—currently referred to as private career schools—and public vocational-technical institutes. Private career schools tend to select students with higher ability and educational attainment than do public vocational-technical institutes (Erickson and others, 1972). Students at private career schools tend to be slightly older than those in collegiate institutions; private career schools also tend to serve a greater proportion of racial minorities. They tend to have a single and well-defined mission "to provide occupational training aimed at placing students in full-time jobs in the shortest time possible" (Youn and Thompson, 1974, p. 77). Because of the emphasis on job placement, these schools have an incentive to respond to changes in market demand and, because of their flexible structure, can add or eliminate programs on the basis of job placement prospects. In short, these schools can serve the training needs of certain allied health occupations quite well. In contrast, the goals of public vocational technical institutes and trade schools may not always be well defined and closely tied to employment needs since these schools are subject to political processes and the regulatory activities of state and local governments.

Programs offered in noncollegiate schools range in length from two weeks to more than two years; programs in private career schools tend to be shorter than those in public schools. The costs of education to students vary by type of program and institution; generally, programs requiring specialized instruction in hospitals and/or expensive equipment cost more than other vocational programs. The lowest-cost institutions for students are public trade and technical schools. In 1972-73, the student costs of education in a proprietary trade and technical institution were $1,233 per nine-month academic year as compared to $1,210 tuition and fees for private two-year colleges, and about $250 tuition and fees for public two-year colleges. Wilms (1974) has argued that attending private career schools is a good investment for the student despite the difference in initial costs because private career school programs are shorter than those in public institutions and the student's losses due to foregone income are therefore lower. Further, private career schools tend to hold the less-advantaged student better than their public counterparts and appear to be more successful in providing jobs for their students of various ethnic backgrounds.

About 1,000 of these postsecondary noncollegiate institutions had one or more allied health programs in 1976. Over four in five were vocational-technical schools or technical institutes (public and private), 10 percent business and commercial schools, 4 percent trade schools, and 1 percent correspondence schools. Sixty-three percent were public, 33 percent were private proprietary or profit-making, and 5 percent were private nonprofit institutions. Although there were more public than private institutions, over half the programs were in the private schools.

Table 13 shows the distribution of 1,059 allied health programs in private career schools (excluding nonprofit ones)

Table 13. Allied Health Programs in Public and Proprietary Noncollegiate Institutions: 1976[a]

	Total		*Public*		*Private Proprietary*	
	Number	*Percent*	*Number*	*Percent*	*Number*	*Percent*
Dental assistant	182	17	62	13	120	20
Dental lab technician	61	6	18	4	43	7
Dental (other)	8	1	2	0+	6	1
EKG/EEG technician	14	1	1	0+	13	2
Medical emergency technician	23	2	18	4	5	1
Medical office assistant	215	20	45	10	170	29
Medical lab assistant	49	5	26	6	23	4
Medical lab (other)	54	5	11	2	43	7
Medical record technician	32	3	6	1	26	4
Mortuary science	9	1	–	–	9	1
Nurse aide	173	16	102	22	71	12
Ophthalmic service	9	1	6	1	3	1
Physician assistant	15	1	6	1	9	1
Psychiatric aide	6	1	3	1	3	1
Radiologic technology	19	2	11	2	8	1
Rehabilitation (including OT, PT assistants)	15	1	9	2	6	1
Respiratory therapy	27	3	13	3	14	2
Surgical technician	38	4	34	7	4	1
Other	110	10	91	20	19	3
Total	1,059	100	464	100	595	100

[a]Excludes 40 programs in non-profit-making private schools, a majority of which were in "nurse aide" or other category.

and public schools for postsecondary vocational training. Four in five allied health programs in private career schools were accounted for by four service categories: medical office assisting (29 percent), dental services (28 percent), nursing aide (12 percent), and medical laboratory services (11 percent). More than half the programs in noncollegiate institutions in the public sector were accounted for by four service categories: nurse aide (22 percent), dental services (18 percent), medical office assistant (10 percent), and surgical technician (7 percent).

From the information available, it is clear that both public and private noncollegiate institutions play an important role in training aide and assistant level personnel in allied health. Because of their short duration and their relatively low costs, such programs make entry into an allied health occupation a possibility for many disadvantaged students. Further, private career schools tend to be highly responsive to employer and community needs. They follow the current practice needs closely and rarely assume a leadership role in terms of what future needs might be—a role more appropriate for programs in academic settings. Further, the sole source of revenue for private career schools is student tuition. This makes the schools dependent upon the success of their graduates in the job market. Therefore, they not only try to place their students after graduation but they also adjust curriculum where necessary, drop programs when demand no longer exists, and add programs as new needs arise. The flexibility of private career schools in adjusting to manpower needs is one of their greatest advantages.

Allied Health Programs in the Armed Forces

Allied health programs in the armed forces are important because they are a source of manpower both for the military and the civilian sector and also because they have successfully initiated educational approaches that may have broad applicability to the civilian programs. For instance, all three branches of the armed forces train health practitioners in multiple competencies, utilize common core curricula, and provide opportunities for relatively smooth career progression. All three services currently use performance-based evaluation techniques. The civilian sector can learn much from techniques employed by the military to simulate clinical experiences.

The Army Enlisted Military Occupational Classification System classifies closely related enlisted positions requiring similar qualifications and performance of duties under generic titles. Each generic title can entail from one to five skills, depending on the type of duty position encompassed. The Army regularly evaluates each enlisted soldier's occupational proficiency.

Although health occupations training courses are given at many facilities across the country, the major facility for the Army is the Academy of Health Sciences at Fort Sam Houston, Texas. The allied medical enrollments in this single facility total about 35,000 students each year, which is equivalent to almost 10 percent of all enrollments in collegiate programs in 1976. There are about 1,700 faculty members, preparing personnel in a wide variety of areas, including health care administration, clinical pastoral education, physical therapy, and medical technology. In 1977, the Army graduated over 16,000 students to provide allied health services.

The Army has successfully implemented a generic curriculum for health occupations, which has been advocated for years but rarely tried in collegiate settings. Completion of the course program for basic medical specialist is a prerequisite for at least twelve other programs in health occupations. The program provides a broad foundation of basic skills and knowledge in many areas, including ambulatory care, environmental medicine, medical records, and emergency medical care. In recent years, Army medical training has undergone a transition from cognitive- to performance-based preparation and evaluation, requiring a greater integration of motor and cognitive skills. On-the-job training has come to play a more significant role. The combination of performance-based education and on-the-job training, coupled with evaluation tests based on skill qualifications, is designed to allow the Army greater ease and accuracy in quality control, as well as more facility in determining job performance for promotional purposes.

The Navy Enlisted Occupational Classification System is designed to allow naval personnel to provide multiple services as required by the limited space aboard ships and submarines. The Navy maintains "occupational standards" by which management may determine Navy requirements for functions performed in health service. The occupational standards are for the minimum level of skill required by a person to perform specified functions. A hospital corpsman is trained to perform multiple functions, and the career ladder for a hospital corpsman ranges from Hospital Apprenticeship through five additional classes to Master Chief Hospital Corpsman, who can perform a wide spectrum of medical functions. Allied health training of naval enlisted personnel is provided at several Navy facilities throughout the United States. In 1977, the Navy programs prepared over 7,500 students in allied health services.

The Air Force system also classifies closely related enlisted positions requiring similar qualifications and performance of duties under generic titles. Each generic title entails up to five skill levels. Skill level career progressions are achieved through a series of academic and on-the-job training experiences.

Although allied health occupational training courses are conducted in Air Force health care facilities across the country and overseas, the majority of academic training is conducted either at the School of Health Care Sciences, Sheppard Air Force Base, Wichita Falls, Texas, or at the School of Aerospace Medicine, Brooks Air Force Base, San Antonio, Texas. Both schools are accredited by the Southern Association of Colleges and Schools. Graduates of these two military schools may also obtain transferable academic credit through the Community College of the Air Force.

The Community College of the Air Force was established by congressional authority and commenced operation in 1972. The college enrolls over 18,000 students annually and offers associate degrees in five areas, including health care sciences. Air Force members enrolled in the college receive degree credit for Air Force courses, on-the-job training, and courses completed at other academic institutions. In 1977, the Air Force trained nearly 12,000 students in allied health services.

All three branches of the armed forces have developed what they believe to be efficient solutions to identifying and training personnel to perform multiple functions, evaluating students on the basis of performance objectives, and providing avenues for career mobility. They have been free to experiment because they are not subject to the numerous forms of regulation and pressures that limit the flexibility of civilian programs. Moreover, their interest in relating educational processes to practice needs derives from the fact that they are both educational institution and employer, and they depend on the persons they prepare to provide health services. Their innovative approaches, such as use of simulated clinical conditions and evaluation of competencies acquired in other settings, should be widely disseminated and discussed for potential application in the collegiate programs.

Of the 30,000 personnel trained in military allied health programs who left the armed forces in 1977, an estimated 10,000 may have found health-related jobs in the civilian sector. The federal government has always been concerned about the assimilation of military-trained personnel into the civilian labor market and has, over the years, funded a number of projects specifically designed to facilitate the utilization of ex-military enlisted personnel: for example, Operation MEDIHC (Military Experience Directed Into Health Careers) and MEDEX (*Medi*cine *Ex*tension). Other efforts to ease the transition of military-trained personnel include those of the Office of Educational Credit of the American Council on Education which, under contract from the Defense Department, has developed, tested, and implemented a program for the evaluation and recognition of military learning acquired not only through formal courses but also through educational experiences such as self-instruction, on-the-job training, and work experience. This information is published and regularly updated by the American Council on Education in the document *Guide to the Evaluation of Educational Experiences in the Armed Services.* Such approaches, which have been designed to relate educational experiences in the military to those in collegiate settings, have broad applicability for evaluating prior learning in allied health education.

Other Settings

The total scope of federally funded allied health education is difficult to estimate because of the wide range of settings in which it is provided other than the principal ones described here. For example, CETA programs under the Department of Labor prepare large numbers of persons to perform relatively routine health functions. The Health Services Administration (Department of Health, Education, and Welfare) operates nine hospitals and supports training activities under the Division of Coast Guard Medical Services, Division of Federal Employer Health, and Division of Health Maintenance Organizations, and in cooperation with the Bureau of Prisons Medical Program, Department of Justice. Some personnel also are prepared in programs operated directly by the states.

There are lessons to be learned from these programs as well. For example, the Coast Guard has demonstrated that physician assistants can be prepared successfully to serve the health needs of persons in remote areas. In many respects, Coast Guard and merchant vessels are comparable to small rural communities on land. The number of persons on board each vessel is not sufficient to warrant the services of a full-time physician, but the officers and crew at sea nevertheless do require medical care. The Public Health Service training program at Staten Island prepares physician assistants to provide the needed medical services, including some surgery, under the radio supervision of physicians based on shore. The success of the arrangement has been attributed to the fact that the physician assistants are trained by the physicians who will supervise them; roles of both are made clear from the outset and, as a result, mutual respect is enhanced.

Schools of Allied Health

The concept of allied health education and the growth of schools of the allied health professions are historically linked. The term *allied health* was first used to describe organizational clusters of health occupations programs in university settings. Both concepts are developed on the assumption that an alliance in education among the numerous health occupations, which separately had little visibility, would build the prestige, strength, and quality of their education. Both concepts were proposed also as a solution to the growing fragmentation of health occupations and the educational processes designed to prepare them for practice; it was argued that an alliance in education would encourage sharing of resources and provide a learning experience conducive to the development of teamwork. The Allied Health Professions Education Subcommittee in 1967 emphasized particularly the provision of a learning environment where individuals who would later work together are prepared together and encouraged "further experimentation with the development of university schools of allied health professions" (Bureau of Health Manpower, 1967, p. 2).

Many early advocates of the allied health education concept were administrators of allied health programs on large medical center campuses. They envisioned the new organizational units of allied health programs on these campuses growing into centers of excellence that could provide allied health students with educational resources on a par with those provided students in medical, dental, nursing, and other health professions schools. They envisioned these centers also fostering research and leadership development. Perhaps their most cherished and idealistic dream was the establishment of peer-level communications and sharing between allied health and other health professions schools, leading to a more integrated health occupations preparation, which would be reflected in practice.

Some argued for establishment of major health science universities that would include schools of medicine, allied health, and other health professions. Pellegrino (1977), a strong proponent of the concept of the university of health sciences, argued that health science centers provide an environment where, theoretically at least, educational and science components can be integrated, multidisciplinary or interdisciplinary arrangement of schools and facilities coordinated, and services articulated to meet community and regional needs.

Growth and Organization of Allied Health Units. During the past decade and a half, many new organizational units have been established in educational institutions throughout the country. A search in the Library of Congress of course catalogues of four-year institutions for the 1978-79 academic year reveals sixty-six schools or colleges of allied health; forty-four have the words allied health in the title and the other twenty-two contain words such as associated health, health-related professions, health technologies, and health sciences. Two thirds of these sixty-six schools are on medical campuses, almost all of which have other health professions schools as well. On some additional campuses, allied health programs are grouped in divisions, departments, and centers. Such units are found in both four-year and two-year institutions, as well as in hospitals and other noncollegiate settings. These different administrative groupings are consistent with the three basic patterns of administrative clusters of allied health programs described by Rosenfeld (1972): (1) a school or college headed by an allied health dean—administratively on a peer level with the medical school; (2) a division or school within the medical school, headed by an allied health director or associate dean; and (3) an administrative unit that serves to coordinate allied health activities housed in various departments. Some variations on these patterns are illustrated by the organizational structures administered by the panel of twenty-three deans and directors of allied health units in academic health centers whom the commission surveyed and used as a sounding board regarding particular study topics. No two campuses are alike. Sixteen of the twenty-three campuses house a school of allied health that is on a peer level with the medical school and that is headed by an allied health dean. On seven campuses, there is no peer school of allied health. Three of these campuses—Baylor, Duke, and Tufts—have an allied health director or associate dean who is concerned with program development and/or coordination but is responsible for few or no course offerings. Three others—Emory, Indiana, and Ohio State—incorporate within the medical school an allied health unit that is headed by an associate dean or director who is responsible for course offerings. In the seventh case, Louisville, some of the allied health programs are offered in a division of allied health that is a separate unit of the health science center but not a "school," as is the medical school.

The institutions represented by these twenty-three administrators are heavily involved in allied health education, with an average of 18 programs and networks of clinical affiliations. The majority report over 50 such affiliations; five report over 150.

Establishing schools of allied health and other administrative clusters was not enough to bring all the programs together. Most respondents, including half the deans of separate allied health schools, describe a spread of programs across various organizational units in their institutions. A comparison of the organizational structures does not reveal any relationship between type of structure and the degree of clustering of allied health programs. One determinant appears to be whether a program was established before or after the allied health unit was formed. The decision to uproot an already established program from, for example, a college of arts and sciences to place it in a new allied health unit is obviously fraught with political implications.

Goals Half Met. How far have the allied health units reached in attaining the ambitious objectives set in the last decade? Have they succeeded in giving allied health programs the same visibility and power as programs for other health occupations? Have they fostered leadership, innovation, and research? Have they promoted communication, collaboration, and cooperation in health sciences education? A major research effort, which was beyond the purview of this commission, would be needed to answer these questions fully. However, the information obtained from the commission's academic health center panel survey—supplemented by review of ASAHP data, literature, and other documents—gives some convincing evidence that the allied health unit has accomplished some objectives but still has obstacles to overcome in reaching others.

Visibility and power: There was consensus among panel members that having an allied health unit, particularly a peer-status school of allied health, increases the visibility and power of allied health programs (as indicated by the ability to obtain financial support and implement programs). However, even separate schools of allied health that are administratively on a peer status with other health professions schools and that may enjoy equal authority, do not have power equal to that of the medical school. The following problems were reported in obtaining resources and developing a strong school of allied health:

- The variety of allied health degrees, as opposed to the single degree in medicine or dentistry, limits visibility and "clout."
- Having programs primarily at the undergraduate level limits power in institutions and reduces research capability—another source of recognition and prestige.
- The low level of federal support to allied health education relative to medicine places the former at a disadvantage. Fewer resources mean less power and less research.
- Lack of a clinical practice plan prohibits faculty from generating some funds for allied health programs and the institution.
- Lack of understanding of allied health services on the part of some physicians and administrators limits recognition of the importance of the programs.

A key factor in the visibility and, to some degree, the power of the allied health unit is the personal relationship between the dean or director of the allied health unit and the vice-president for health affairs. Some observers have hypothesized that the service orientation of allied health programs reduces the prestige of these programs, particularly if they are housed in research-oriented campuses, or if the medical school is research oriented. Many of the medical schools in the same health science centers as the respondents are also service oriented, but where differences in orientation exist, they do not seem to result in any problems. One dean comments that, while the allied health school is trying to develop a research capability similar to that of the medical school, the medical school is trying to develop a service capability like that of the allied health school—a reminder that a service orientation should not be denigrated.

Leadership, innovation, and research: There is no question about the significant role allied health schools and other administrative units have played in leadership development, innovation, and research. Although relatively new, many have developed model programs for advanced education; some of the incentives for such programs, particularly in teaching and administration, have come from the W. K. Kellogg Foundation's Allied Health Instructional Personnel grants. These allied health units have also stimulated some scholarly activity; about half the articles published in the *Journal of Allied Health* since it was introduced in 1972 were authored by one or more persons employed in such a unit, and a cursory examination of books and monographs related to allied health shows a similar pattern.

It is difficult to determine to what extent these contributions can be attributed to organizational settings and to what extent to the individuals who are attracted to such settings. Respondents in the commission's survey panel believe that health science settings are more likely than other settings to attract research funds and stimulate research and innovation. However, they do not believe that any particular administrative organization is more advantageous than others for these activities, which are seen as more contingent upon faculty qualifications and achievements.

Moreover, the level of research activity could be substantially increased. Only half the respondents report that basic research on education or practice in allied health professions is currently being conducted by many of their faculty. The major obstacles are lack of funding, especially for basic research, lack of laboratory space and equipment, lack of interest on the part of tenured faculty, limited faculty time and capabilities, and lack of graduate programs and students. Suggestions to increase research activities include hiring new faculty with research capabilities and experience, providing in-service training, collaborating with basic science departments, and, finally, adopting a reward system for research.

With respect to leadership development, respondents do see definite advantages in the separate allied health school. They believe that an environment in which allied health and medical faculty and administrators are peers provides a strong role model for allied health students and promotes a sense of self-worth.

Communication, collaboration, and cooperation: One of the obvious advantages of being housed in a health science center is the potential for allied health students and faculty to benefit from interaction with students and faculty from various health professions schools. There are different avenues for interaction: interdisciplinary activities in didactic education, interdisciplinary activities in clinical education, research projects, and committee work.

Most frequently reported cases of interaction between and within health professions schools involve interdisciplinary activities where students enrolled in different allied health programs are taught together in a classroom. Allied health faculty and medical faculty also occasionally work together. Interdisciplinary activities involving other health professions students or faculty are less frequently reported.

In clinical education, the allied health and medical faculty are more likely to work together than allied health and other faculty. Allied health and medical students, and to a lesser degree, allied health students and those from other health professions schools have some opportunity to share clinical experience. Research activities result in some interaction between allied health and medical faculty but involve very few students. Committee work and other administrative tasks provide interaction for both faculty and students.

Overall, however, most respondents feel that not enough interaction takes place among faculty or among students. Obstacles to interaction, in the opinion of respondents, include rigidity and time constraints, lack of control over clinical education, large class size, physical separation and distance between schools, and negative attitudes and lack of interest of faculty.

In summary, the concept of separate allied health schools and of allied health units in health science centers is endorsed as a viable one by most of our respondents. Some of the promises held by such schools have been fulfilled; others will seem to fall short. Although the idea of clustering programs under one administrative unit is a solid one, perhaps it is not the administrative organization that is most important but the proximity of programs with commonalities in interest and knowledge base, and the willingness of administrators and educators in these programs to collaborate and share.

Some interaction is already taking place. But what seems to be lacking is a commitment to placing community interests above those of individual programs. Partially, the lack of commitment may be due to problems arising from accreditation processes that treat each program as a separate entity, and, partially, it results from a lack of recognition of commonalities in curriculum. Mutual appreciation and collaboration among allied health program directors, on the one hand, and between allied health and other health groups, on the other, will accelerate the development of a common knowledge base in all health fields and will reduce the unnecessary duplication of effort, making the educational process for all more cost-effective.

Method in Apparent Madness

In spite of the tremendous diversity of allied health education with respect to educational settings and levels, the widely held belief that the allied health scene is characterized by chaos is simply not true. Without a doubt, allied health education is growing and changing constantly, and it is so far-ranging that attempts to define its limits and measure its components in terms of total number of programs, total number of students, or total output have been so far futile. However, there is considerably more method in this apparent madness than meets the eye. The constant growth and change in education are necessary responses to the growth and change in what is probably the most dynamic industry in the United States—the health industry. The wide range of occupational preparation programs in different disciplines and at different levels corresponds to the diverse health service needs and to the broad differences between health occupations in knowledge and skill requirements and responsibilities. It would not be appropriate today for all health occupations to be prepared at the same educational level.

Moreover, the distribution of educational programs in different settings appears rational. There is considerably less overlap in the activities and objectives of different program settings than is generally believed. Of the 139 occupational categories for which there were collegiate programs, nearly 57 percent were found only in four-year colleges or only in two-year colleges. Programs in four-year colleges tended to be at the therapist and technologist or higher levels, whereas the programs in two-year colleges tended to be at the assistant and technician level. Of the 82 allied health occupations included in hospital-based programs, all but 8 had counterparts in collegiate settings. However, only 6 occupations had a large number of programs in both hospital and collegiate settings: medical technologist, dietitian, radiologic technologist, emergency medical technician, operating room technician, and nurse aide.

As a general pattern, an occupation is likely to have hospital-based educational programs if it requires less than a bachelor's degree for entry, its practitioners are employed chiefly in hospital settings, and/or a large component of its training requires expensive equipment. Hospital-based programs for occupations generally taught at the baccalaureate level in academic settings almost always include some postsecondary education as a prerequisite for entry. For example, some prior collegiate education is required in all hospital-based programs for medical technologists, cytotechnologists, medical records administrators, nutritionists, clinical pastoral counselors, and a variety of therapists and nurse specialists.

The degree of overlap among collegiate, noncollegiate, and hospital programs is more difficult to determine because of differences in program titles. It appears that most of the programs in noncollegiate settings are also given in hospitals or collegiate settings; however, the major mission of these settings—to provide short-term preparation for entry-level jobs—is well reflected in the types of programs offered. Unless more information is available to make quality comparisons among these programs, it is difficult to assess the impact of overlap where it does exist. Clearly, some programs are firmly entrenched in one type of setting. Others are given in more than one setting. A degree of overlap between collegiate and noncollegiate settings for occupations at the assistant and technician levels may be valuable for providing adequate access to allied health programs and a variety of optional routes to employment. Students interested in short-term training directly applicable to employment may find hospital or noncollegiate programs preferable; those interested in a broader education and with some expectation of pursuing further formal education may choose collegiate programs.

Some observers have expressed concern about overlap in educational degree levels, believing that, in many instances, programs for the same occupation are offered at different degree levels. The number of occupations with which this overlap phenomenon is associated is not great: Four in ten allied health occupations with collegiate programs were prepared only at the baccalaureate level and three in ten only at the associate degree or lower division certificate level (see Tables 14 and 15). However, the overlap that does exist may indeed be problematic. An examination of objectives, prerequisites, and course offerings of programs at different award levels in four occupations indicates that some of the programs leading to higher degrees are geared to higher levels of practice, but others are not. Thus graduates with different degrees enter the market for the same jobs. This phenomenon is likely to create confusion and problems for employers and graduates alike when degrees are used as a criterion for employment, as is the case for most health occupations today. When different degree levels are justified by practice requirements or other valid considerations, it is imperative for students to be given accurate information and effective counseling so that they choose the most appropriate program to meet their own objectives.

Table 14. Occupations for Which Collegiate Preparation Is at the Baccalaureate Level or Higher

Baccalaureate Programs Only	*Certificate and Baccalaureate Programs*	*Baccalaureate and Graduate Programs*	*Certificate, Baccalaureate, and Graduate Programs*	*Graduate Programs Only*
Allied health educator	Specialist in blood bank technology	Health care administrator	Occupational therapist	Biostatistician
Microbiology technologist	Medical technologist	Dietitian/nutritionist	Biomedical engineer	Audiologist
Community/public health educator	Sanitarian aide	Nutritionist		Speech pathologist
Dietitian	Orthoptist	Environmental engineer		
Medical communication specialist		Sanitarian		
Medical illustrator		Health educator		
Medical record administrator		Occupational therapist		
Manual arts therapist		Physical therapist		
Corrective therapist		Art therapist		
Rehabilitation therapy technician		Recreational therapist		
Music therapist		Medical/psychiatric social worker		
Speech pathologist (pre-master's)		Rehabilitation counselor		
Speech pathologist/audiologist (pre-master's)		Speech pathologist/audiologist		
		Health physicist		

Note: This table includes only those occupations for which 5 or more collegiate programs were identified. Occupations listed under a combination of degree levels had at least 2 collegiate programs at each degree level in the combination.

Source: ASAHP 1976 Collegiate Inventory.

Table 15. Occupations for Which Collegiate Preparation May Be at the Associate Degree Level or Less

Lower Division Certificate Programs Only	*Associate Degree Programs Only*	*Associate and Certificate Programs*	*Associate and Baccalaureate Programs*	*Associate, Certificate, and Baccalaureate Programs*	*Associate, Baccalaureate, and Graduate Programs*	*Certificate, Associate, and Graduate Programs*	*Certificate, Associate, Baccalaureate, and Graduate Programs*
Unit clerk	Cardiopulmonary technician	Medical office assistant	Long-term care administrator	Biomedical engineer technician	Health care assistant administrator	Alcohol/drug abuse specialist	Community health worker
Medical lab assistant	Ophthalmic optician	Medical/dental secretary	Environmental health technician	Cytotechnologist	School health educator		
Dietetic assistant	Physical therapy assistant	Histologic technician	Mental health technologist	Dental hygienist	Industrial hygienist		
Ambulance attendant	Child care worker	Dental assistant	Orthotist/prosthetist	Human services technologist/technician	Public health practitioner, NEC		
Respiratory therapy technician		Dental technician	Physician assistant/specialty	Mental health associate/technician/assistant			
Homemaker/home health aide		Dietetic technician	Rehabilitation counselor aide	Nuclear medicine technologist/technician			
Ophthalmic laboratory technician		Emergency medical technician		Geriatric care worker			
		Environmental engineering assistant		Physician assistant (primary care)			
		Electroencephalographic technologist/technician					

(continued on next page)

Table 15 (Continued)

Lower Division Certificate Programs Only	*Associate Degree Programs Only*	*Associate and Certificate Programs*	*Associate and Baccalaureate Programs*	*Associate, Certificate, and Baccalaureate Programs*	*Associate, Baccalaureate, and Graduate Programs*	*Certificate, Associate, and Graduate Programs*	*Certificate, Associate, Baccalaureate, and Graduate Programs*
		Medical record technician		Radiologic technologist/technician			
		Medical transcriptionist		Respiratory therapist			
		Mental retardation aide					
		Psychiatric technician					
		Operating room technician					
		Ophthalmic dispenser					
		Optometric assistant/technician					
		Occupational therapy assistant					
		Medical lab technician					
		Radiation therapy technologist/technician					

Note: This table includes only those occupations for which five or more collegiate programs were identified. Occupations listed under a combination of degree levels had at least two collegiate programs at each degree level in the combination.

Source: ASAHP 1976 Collegiate Inventory.

V

Toward Educational Alliances

In 1968, Mase (1968) proposed "three C's for allied health education: communication, collaboration, and cooperation." The need for a genuine alliance in health service—stressed repeatedly in Chapters Two and Three—has been and continues to be equally important for the education of health manpower. A decade ago, collaboration was considered important primarily for its impact on the quality of education, but today it is seen as valuable, if not essential, for meeting organizational and administrative challenges in an era of austerity.

This chapter examines promising collaborative approaches between and within institutions which show promise for meeting the goals of quality, cost containment, continuity in educational process, and, in some cases, increasing access to allied health education. Generally, collaborative models cannot be transferred intact from one setting to another but must be tailored to the needs and environments of different institutional settings. Moreover, the success of any approach or model may depend on many factors, including support from top administrators at the institutional level and such intangibles as the capabilities and personalities of those directly involved. To date, there are no reported research efforts designed explicitly to determine whether one type of collaborative effort is more effective than another. However, the information available is suggestive of some useful patterns.

Reaching Out: Collaboration Between Educational Institutions

The concept of collaboration among institutions is not a novel one for allied health. From the start, collegiate programs have entered into agreements with clinical facilities providing practicum experiences for students. The 1967 subcommittee report reflected the enthusiasm of allied health educators for collaborative arrangements and coordinated planning. These efforts were aimed primarily at upgrading the quality of education and meeting increasing manpower needs. One recommendation called for "regional, state, and community-wide planning for development of educational programs, including strengthened liaison between junior and senior colleges and medical centers" (Bureau of Health Manpower, 1967, p. 2). Since that time, coordinated planning mechanisms have become widespread, and voluntary collaborative arrangements for didactic as well as clinical education are commonplace in allied health education. Some of the different types of voluntary collaborative arrangements involving didactic education are described here. Although quality and manpower considerations remain important, a major impetus for coordinated planning and collaboration today is efficient utilization of resources.

The Cooperative Movement: Federal Impetus. Collaboration in allied health education has not occurred in isolation but parallels the growth of the voluntary cooperative movement, one of the most significant trends in postsecondary education during the past decade. It has been impossible to count accurately the ever increasing number of collaborative arrangements —voluntary or statutory—that have occurred within colleges and universities in the United States. In 1974, the number was estimated at 10,000 and is probably well over that figure today (Conners and others, 1974).

Although the cooperative movement has developed most

rapidly since the mid sixties, its beginnings are usually traced back to the establishment of university centers at Claremont, California, and Atlanta, Georgia, more than half a century ago. After World War II, GI Bill enrollments created a demand for education that higher education institutions were unable to meet. Collaboration was a major solution to the problem of limited resources. The establishment of the Southern Regional Education Board, in 1949, and the Western Interstate Compact for Higher Education and the New England Board of Higher Education, both in 1953, was followed by a series of state and regional agreements, which furthered interest in institutional collaboration.

The federal government has played a major role in these activities. The Higher Education Facilities Act of 1963 (P.L. 88-204) brought national attention to the idea of cooperation; the Higher Education Act of 1965 (P.L. 89-329) authorized grants "to pay part of the cost of planning, developing, and carrying out cooperative arrangements which show promise as effective measures for strengthening the academic programs and the administration of developing institutions."

With the establishment of the Regional Medical Programs (RMP) through the Heart Disease, Cancer, and Stroke Amendments of 1965 (P.L. 89-239), the federal government turned its attention more specifically to cooperative arrangements for educating health personnel. In 1972, supplemental funds were provided under the RMP program for the development of area health consortia; subsequently, 105 consortia were established for the primary purpose of relating educational programs to the health needs of the community. RMPs were phased out in 1974 with the creation of new state and local structures for health planning.

Another significant stimulus for collaboration was the provision of health manpower education initiative awards for the establishment of area health education centers (AHECs) (Comprehensive Health Manpower Training Act, P.L. 92-157). Since 1972, the fifteen AHEC projects have received funds to link schools of medicine, university health science centers, and other institutions in medically underserved areas for the purpose of improving educational resources. Additional funds were provided to AHECs under the Health Professions Assistance Act of 1976 (P.L. 94-484) "for the purpose of improving the distribution, supply, quality, utilization, and efficiency of health personnel in the health services delivery system and for the purpose of encouraging the regionalization of educational responsibilities of health professions schools." P.L. 94-484 (Section 796) also authorized project grants and contracts for "planning, developing, and evaluating projects to establish a regional or state system for the coordination of education and training at various levels for allied health personnel and nurses within and among educational institutions and their clinical affiliates for the purpose of assuring that allied health and nurse manpower needs of the region are substantially met."

Growing State and Regional Coordination. Concurrently with increasing federal interest in educational planning and management effectiveness, state agencies began a closer scrutiny of educational growth. The 1202 Commissions, established by the Education Amendments of 1972 (P.L. 92-318), have expanded the scope of their functions. Most states routinely review requests for new programs, and at least twenty states now have extended the review process to existing programs. In 1975, thirty-five states had completed long-range planning for postsecondary education; by 1976, twenty-eight states had some responsibility for planning private as well as public education (Borak and Berdahl, 1978).

State planning activities focus primarily on accountability and efficiency through program review and incentives for interinstitutional cooperation. The new catchword is regionalism, which refers to coordinated planning of resource utilization in a given geographic area. This may be either a portion of a state or an area that includes all or part of more than one state. Of the ninety-eight regionalization activities identified by Martorana and Nespoli, about two thirds covered within-state regions and the remainder crossed state lines (Martorana and Nespoli, 1978).

The National Health Planning and Resources Development Act of 1974 (P.L. 93-641) established new state agencies to deal with health planning, with the major purpose of containing rising health care costs. The approximately two hundred Health Systems Agencies (HSAs) are required to draw up Health Service Plans and Annual Implementation Plans for their health service areas. These plans must include supply and requirement projections and specify manpower planning activities. The Statewide Health Coordinating Councils (SHCCs) then review and coordinate the plans for the HSAs within each state. The State Health Planning Development Agency (SHPDA) has the final responsibility for developing a comprehensive state health plan. In a background study prepared for this commission, Commissioner Darrel Mase (1978) concluded that these new health planning agencies have as yet rarely played an active role in planning or coordination of allied health education. However, as these agencies become increasingly effective in carrying out their cost-containment mandate, they can be expected to focus more directly on health occupations preparation.

Because of their rapid and seemingly unplanned growth, allied health programs are a prime target for state planning initiatives. Planning committees for allied health education have been established in a number of states, within higher education boards. In an effort to promote better coordination of the activities of the various agencies involved in health manpower planning, the Bureau of Health Manpower, Health Resources Administration (Department of Health, Education, and Welfare) awarded contracts to twenty-two states to develop formal and informal linkages among producers and users of health manpower, state agencies, professional associations, and other involved groups. Currently, the Southern Regional Education Board is working with state higher education agencies in the South to develop mechanisms for regional coordination of allied health education. Clearly, coordinated planning at the regional, state, and local levels—through voluntary or regulated efforts—will continue to be an increasingly important factor for allied health education in the future.

Types of Interinstitutional Collaboration. Although consortium arrangements—reflecting major collaborative efforts at the institutional level—would seem a natural starting point for the examination of cooperation within allied health education, available data indicate that at present this is not the case. In September 1978, the commission staff surveyed 114 established voluntary academic consortia and all state agencies responsible for postsecondary collegiate and vocational technical education. The results show that few established consortia are involved in allied health education. Most are worked out between institutions on a per program basis rather than as part of a master interinstitutional plan.

Collaborative arrangements in allied health are generally guided by one or more of the following purposes: (1) special manpower purposes—for example, to meet program needs of rural areas; (2) resource utilization purposes—for example, to meet program needs for expensive equipment and facilities and to avoid unnecessary duplication of resources; (3) student-oriented purposes—for example, to provide opportunities for the transition from one program to another without unnecessary duplication of learning and to enable students to receive academic recognition of achievement.

Collaboration for special manpower purposes: Collaborative arrangements between institutions have been initiated in order to supply manpower for geographical areas where small numbers of new graduates are needed on a continuing basis or where production requirements are of short-term duration. Institutions also have collaborated to meet national or regional needs for personnel in occupations that serve an important role in the health system but for which demand in any geographical area is limited to a small number.

A major concern has been the provision of adequate manpower to medically underserved rural areas. One collaborative model for meeting these needs, the *urban-rural linkage model,* is based on the assumption that students from remote areas are more likely to stay in their home community to practice if they complete some of their occupational preparation in the home community. This model links remote educational institutions with an urban institution that has substantial existing resources for instruction in health fields. Students complete part of their education in the large urban complex and part in their home institution. By providing part of the program in the home community, out-migration is reduced. In addition, there is some potential for attracting urban students into the rural underserved areas by exposing them to the health service environment in these areas. The remote institutions offer courses of relatively generic nature, which do not tax their educational resources.

The best-known urban-rural collaboration project of this kind, and one that has served as a model for other efforts, is the Junior College-Regional Technical Institute Linkage Program (JC-RTI) in Alabama. This highly successful arrangement links twenty-four rural two-year colleges in the state with the Regional Technical Institute (RTI) of the School of Community and Allied Health of the University of Alabama at Birmingham for allied health education in fourteen specialty areas. Initial funding support was provided by the Alabama Regional Medical Program, followed by a five-year grant from the W. K. Kellogg Foundation. The linkage arrangement affords students from rural areas the opportunity to learn in a major medical center that has a wide variety of medical clinics and more than 2,000 patient beds. Students attend the two-year colleges for approximately one year of nontechnical prerequisite courses, then transfer to RTI for the second year of technical study and clinical experience. The final eight to ten weeks of technical training are arranged with clinical affiliates in the students' home communities. The relatively high proportion of graduates who practice in their home communities is attributed to the fact that students study in Birmingham for just one year and return to the home community for the final period.

The JC-RTI program is now being linked across state lines to other programs. For example, Florida Junior College at Jacksonville is cooperating with the University of Alabama for a linkage program for two allied health disciplines. The Southern Arizona Regional Allied Health Education Linkage Program (SARAHELP), also based on the JC-RTI model, was established in 1975. This program was designed to address health manpower needs by developing educational linkages between urban Pima County and sparsely populated counties in the state.

The Pima County Community College in Tucson houses a

number of allied health programs, has fully equipped laboratories, and maintains clinical affiliations with the University of Arizona Medical Center, greater metropolitan Tucson and Phoenix hospitals, and health care centers in Cochise and Yuma counties. Through SARAHELP, students take up to one year of liberal arts, pretechnical, and introductory technical study at their home community college, followed by one year of technical and clinical education in the Pima County Community College District. Some of the clinical training may occur within the student's home community. Administrators of SARAHELP believe that the linkage system permits students to receive the best technical training available in the Southern Arizona region, avoids costly duplication of college-based programs, and encourages students to return to their home communities for service. To date, about one third of SARAHELP graduates have returned to their rural communities to practice. For those who do not return, the program meets a secondary objective: to provide career opportunities to persons in areas where such opportunities would otherwise be limited.

Similarly, two community colleges in sparsely populated areas of Florida—Lake Sumpter Community College in Leesburg and Seminole Community College in Sanford—have formal agreements to send a specified number of students who have successfully completed the first year of study in nursing and allied health programs to Valencia Community College in Orlando, where they complete their requirements for an associate degree. As in the JC-RTI and SARAHELP examples, neither of the two outlying community colleges can justify the costs of full programs for allied health occupations based on the needs of their service area. Moreover, the clinical facilities in urban Orlando are unmatched in the two rural communities.

The most geographically extended urban-rural linkage system for health occupations education is the Washington, Alaska, Montana, and Idaho Consortium (WAMI), which comprises one medical center and one health science center at the University of Washington, the state universities of the other three states, and Washington State University (which is located in the somewhat isolated eastern part of the state). Thus far, the consortium arrangement has been limited to medical students, but plans are under way to include some allied health occupations in the future. Students selected into WAMI from the three other states and from Washington State University receive the first year of education on their home campuses and then go to the University of Washington for the next three years. As in the JC-RTI and SARAHELP systems, students spend their final year in a clinical practicum in their home area, in the hope that they will develop local practice ties and be encouraged to remain. In the WAMI case, with its vast territorial coverage, the "local area" may encompass an entire state. Essential to the success of WAMI is an effective communications system. Through the use of a satellite providing two-way audiovisual communication, faculty from the University of Washington Medical Center can give lectures and conduct seminars with students 1,000 miles away; they also can work closely with faculty at different sites for planning and administration.

A ten-member consortium, operating since 1973 in Western Washington state, illustrates the applicability of the urban-rural linkage model to hospitals. The hub of this Health Services Consortium is an urban medical center in Seattle, which is linked with smaller hospitals in nine communities in the region. The linkage provides the outlying communities with much-needed health training capabilities and continuing education opportunities. Start-up funds were provided by the W. K. Kellogg Foundation for a three-year period during which the program reported substantial progress toward achieving both these objectives.

Also promising for meeting special manpower needs, but rarely applied in allied health education, is the *short-term program collaborative model.* Winthrop College in South Carolina found that there was a demand for a bachelor's degree nurse program but expected the demand to be of short-term duration. The college recognized that the high start-up costs would not be warranted for a program of a temporary nature. Moreover, terminating a collegiate program that is no longer needed is no easy matter. Therefore, an agreement was worked out for the Medical University of South Carolina to set up and run a program at Winthrop College for the four- or five-year period until student demand ended. Start-up costs were below those usually associated with a program of this nature because of the resources provided by the medical center.

A different model for meeting special manpower needs is the *intensive training center approach* used by Oak Ridge Associated Universities (ORAU), headquartered at Oak Ridge, Tennessee. This center helps to meet multistate needs for health physicists, an occupational category for which the number of openings in any given location is likely to be small. The intensive five-week twenty-hour program prepares twenty-four students at a time. Faculty, who are drawn from ORAU's forty-five member colleges and universities from all over the United States, also benefit from the interaction with colleagues and from contact with a research-oriented environment.

A fourth model is the *student exchange contract.* On a large scale, this model is exemplified by the interstate contract. The Health Professions Contract Program, which is part of the New England Regional Student Program of the New England Board of Higher Education, is a case in point. By agreement, each state can make use of occupational preparation programs in other New England states by reserving a specified number of places in these programs and contracting with students regarding financial support and obligations. In the 1977-78 academic year, the six New England states enrolled 263 undergraduate students in physical and occupational therapy programs at Boston, Northeastern, and Tufts universities. Because of the high educational costs and concern over lack of incentive to return to the home state, three states now require that participating students either repay the educational costs or provide equivalent services.

Similarly, the Academic Common Market program developed by the Southern Regional Education Board allows the fourteen participating states to arrange for qualified residents to enroll in programs in other states on an instate tuition basis. In 1979, for the first time, undergraduate programs in a number of allied health occupations were offered in the Academic Common Market in addition to graduate degree programs. The

Southern Regional Education Board believes that this interstate sharing arrangement reduces unnecessary duplication of educational resources while increasing the access of participating states to allied health education.

On a smaller scale, student exchange agreements may be developed by two states for a single purpose. For example, the School of Allied Health Professions at Louisiana State University and the School of Health Related Professions at the University of Mississippi exchange students in occupational therapy and medical records. The agreement allows five Mississippi residents to enter the occupational therapy program at Louisiana State University's School of Health Related Professions (where they are treated as Louisiana residents) and, in return, allows five Louisiana residents to enter the Mississippi program in medical records.

Collaboration for resource utilization purposes: Numerous collaborative arrangements have been developed for the purpose of avoiding unnecessary duplication of allied health education resources and for making the most efficient use of existing resources. These arrangements may be multipurpose peer arrangements, bilateral peer arrangements, or paternalistic arrangements.

Among the large-scale *multipurpose peer arrangements* is the Virginia Health Education Consortium, one of the few formal consortia established exclusively for collaboration in educating health personnel. The member institutions serve a diverse student population and include two traditionally black institutions, one highly selective residential institution, and a large urban regional university. The three initial goals of the consortium were: (1) to minimize duplication, (2) to relate health education programs, regional hospitals, and institutions of higher education into an operational framework, and (3) to disburse resources in the most efficient and appropriate way.

Two types of collaborative activities are essential components of this consortium: In cooperative programs, individual institutions give separate degrees and formulate written agreements to share staff, facilities, faculty, and coursework. In joint programs, a single degree is offered and participating institutions provide approximately equal parts of the education. In addition, when one member institution establishes a program, openings are reserved for students from other member institutions.

The collaboration has led to expanded resources for all participants and has provided greater career opportunities to the students in the traditionally black institutions. In a presentation to the commission, Donald F. Taylor, Director of Health Services at Norfolk State College, pointed out that lack of support for traditionally black institutions resulted, for many, in a curriculum that prepared graduates only "to preach or to teach." The College now is able to avail itself of equipment and facilities it could not otherwise afford to prepare students for allied health careers.

Another general purpose consortium, in Charleston, includes the Medical University of South Carolina, two public four-year colleges, a private four-year liberal arts and teachers college, a public two-year college, and the South Carolina Department of Wildlife and Marine Resources. This consortium arrangement facilitates communication among member institutions, resource sharing, and student exchange. Currently, the Medical University and Trident Technical College collaborate in offering allied health programs. The Medical University is also helping another consortium member, the College of Charleston, build a medical illustration program onto the capabilities of the existing drafting department.

Louisiana State University makes maximum use of faculty and administrative resources by arrangement between campuses. The allied health programs at Shreveport and New Orleans all operate under the aegis of department heads and a dean, all based in New Orleans. Faculty and clinical-site management personnel on the two campuses are frequently exchanged, not only for specific program needs but also to develop the expertise and mutual understanding of these individuals.

Bilateral cooperative arrangements between individual programs are usually designed to improve quality and/or reduce costs of education by pooling complementary resources. These arrangements often involve institutions of different types and control, one of which may have better technical and/or clinical facilities than the other. Baylor College of Medicine (a private institution) has a collaborative arrangement with Texas A & M University and the University of Houston (both public institutions) to offer a graduate program in allied health teacher education and administration. Baylor College of Medicine also has a cooperative agreement to offer a baccalaureate program in nuclear medical technology with the University of Houston (public) and Houston Baptist University (private).

Also in Texas, Navarro Junior College and El Centro College, a public two-year institution, have joint programs in nursing and radiologic technology. Students are registered at both institutions, and faculty take part in the activities of both campuses. The collaboration began after Texas issued a moratorium on additional registered nurse programs; El Centro had already been approved to offer such a program but saw advantages in using the clinical facilities and basic science capabilities of Navarro.

Whereas the Navarro-El Centro arrangement exemplifies *peer-type* collaboration, bilateral arrangements in allied health often involve a *paternalistic relationship* between a medical center and local colleges. For example, two community colleges in Florida use the J. Hillis Miller Health Center of the University of Florida as their clinical campus; the programs are administered by a clinical education committee at the University of Florida. Other arrangements mentioned earlier, such as the JC-RTI linkage system, also involve paternalistic relationships.

In general, academic health centers have assumed a responsibility for providing educational services that extend beyond the limits of their own campus. The commission's 1978 survey of allied health schools and other administrative units in twenty-three academic health centers shows that nearly two thirds offer programs in allied health leading to a degree or certificate given by another institution.

Collaboration for student-oriented purposes: Any arrangement developed to improve the quality of education benefits the student; however, some arrangements are specifically designed to facilitate student progress and career development.

A field as diverse and heterogeneous as allied health—with its multilevel occupations, educational settings ranging from traditional classrooms to health care delivery settings, and its extensive experiential learning component—presents problems of student mobility that have only begun to be addressed through institutional arrangements.

Some states have arrangements between the public two-year colleges and four-year colleges and universities which facilitate the progress of students from preprofessional programs to professional programs or from professional programs in two-year colleges to four-year college programs for advanced specialty training or extension of skills into teaching and administration. More problematic, however, is any transition of students from lower to higher occupational levels within an occupational field. In only a few instances (for example, medical laboratory sciences) has movement from one occupational level to another been sufficiently worked out so that it is viewed as a natural transition.

A model program in medical laboratory sciences, developed in northern Illinois, facilitates the transition from the medical laboratory technician level to the technologist level. This program enables students who complete accredited medical laboratory technician (MLT) programs in community colleges to continue studies toward a baccalaureate degree in medical technology (MT) at the University of Illinois, without loss of time or repetition of learning. Curriculum sequencing in the University of Illinois program was rearranged to include arts and sciences in year one, basic medical technology in year two, continued arts and sciences in year three, and advanced medical technology in year four. The first two years correspond to the content of accredited MLT programs in the state; the last two years complete the required MT preparation. Other special features include the recognition of the clinical portion of the MLT programs and the use of validation examinations, which were developed by a statewide committee of MLT and MT educators.

Transfer remains a major problem for many students in higher education. To date, thirty-nine states have developed policies to ease the transfer of credits from a two-year to a four-year institution; however, these policies generally relate to students whose two-year college major was in arts and sciences rather than occupational preparation. Transfer of credit from such occupational programs (which often are designated as non-transfer or terminal) is still problematic (Holmstrom and Bisconti, 1974). It is especially difficult for students to transfer from noncollegiate to collegiate settings, with credit awarded for prior learning, because criteria and procedures for evaluating learning that takes place outside a collegiate setting are not well developed for allied health education. The Airlie House Conference on Transfer recommended the establishment and publication of "criteria for assigning credit to nontraditional educational experiences (for example, military, technical, vocational, experiential, industrial, cooperative, independent study, internship, and related modes of education) through nontraditional evaluation procedures such as challenge exams, as well as the College Level Examination Program, the American Council on Education's Office on Educational Credit, and other national testing and evaluation programs" (Association Transfer Group, 1974, p. 2). Although some progress in this direction has been made for postsecondary education in general, there is very little evidence of the use of nontraditional evaluation procedures in allied health education.

Transfer between disciplines is also extremely difficult. It seems clear that a first step toward facilitating transfer between disciplines in the same institution or in different institutions must be genuine recognition of and appreciation for commonalities in functions, continuities in skills and knowledge base, and shared objectives, values, and goals.

In summary, the variety of successful collaborative arrangements reported here attests to the vigor of the allied health field. Although designed to meet specific institutional and regional or local needs, they appear to have wider applicability for allied health education. Lessons can be learned from more in-depth study and broader sharing of the experiences of those who have already tried such arrangements.

Learning Together: Collaboration Between Disciplines

Allied health education often occurs in highly insulated and isolated units within institutions. Programs may be planned, established, administered, and operated as if they bore little relationship to any surrounding educational activities. In large part, this isolation results from the fact that allied health programs are designed to prepare students for specific occupational roles. Program content is largely governed by essentials determined by separate professional groups, and the processes are assessed separately by accreditation teams. Moreover, accreditation standards frequently require separate administrators for each allied health program. As a result, small turfdoms have sometimes grown up, and protection of turf has become a principal barrier to collaboration. Administrators of allied health programs in a particular institution may not be aware of the commonalities between their own programs and others. They may be unaware that some of their own courses, particularly in basic sciences, essentially duplicate those of other programs.

Because allied health disciplines are frequently seen as "vocational," they may be assigned a lower status than that of liberal arts majors. Failure to recognize the extremely rigorous course content in much of allied health education can lead to further isolation from the mainstream of campus life. In addition, medicine and nursing programs often show little enthusiasm for collaboration with allied health programs, either because their own curriculum is also tightly structured or because of misconceptions regarding the quality of the allied health disciplines.

Despite these barriers, there are numerous examples of collaborative activities in allied health education involving joint planning and the sharing of resources and learning experiences. These activities are based on several premises. First is the premise that use of existing resources is more efficient than duplication of resources on the same campus. The second premise is that joint planning and sharing of experiences can lead to more effective educational processes. A third premise is that sharing learning experiences promotes the collaboration in practice essential in today's complex health delivery system. The value of the allied health concept for education lies in the assumption that there exists, among this diverse group, a commonality of objectives as well as a sense of teamwork, and implicit in this is the expectation that there is or should be a sharing of learning experiences (Hamburg, 1969).

Interdisciplinary Processes. From the 1960s, when the allied health education concept was first widely promoted, until today the most discussed form of intrainstitutional collaboration has been interdisciplinary education. In 1967, the Allied Health Education Subcommittee recommended "further experimentation with the development of interdisciplinary health personnel education centers, including university schools of allied health" (Bureau of Health Manpower, 1967, p. 2).

There is general agreement that objectives of interdisciplinary education include the following: (1) preparation of the health professional student to deliver coordinated health care; (2) development of a common philosophical framework for sharing of values and goals; (3) development of mutual respect among various members of the health care team; (4) development of willingness to share responsibility for planning and delivery of health care with other health professionals; (5) orientation of the student to the various health occupational roles in order to facilitate cross-disciplinary communication and planning of health care; (6) development of a common language among health professionals; and (7) promotion and demonstration of the delivery of team health care (Jacobsen, 1977, p. 107).

Interdisciplinary education should be conceptualized as a process, allowing interaction among students and trainees from different health occupations for the purposes of learning, problem solving, patient care, and the like. It implies much more than the process of teaching educational content common to more than one occupation or a teaching situation utilizing faculty from more than one discipline, as has been suggested (Pellegrino, 1977, p. 9).

The process of interdisciplinary education involves many models. In a comprehensive paper prepared for this commission,

Connelly (1978, p. 33) identified four major models of interdisciplinary activities currently in use in allied health education: (1) common issue, (2) case presentation, (3) research team, and (4) patient care team.

The *common issue model* requires the development of course material that is used by more than one discipline in classroom settings. Lectures and small group discussion focus on a common issue, such as ethics in the health care system. Examples include the University of Nevada at Reno project where an integrated curriculum from freshman through professional school was prepared for students from medicine, nursing, medical technology, physical therapy, health education, and speech pathology and audiology. Another example is Kellogg Community College's "Health Technology 10" Integrated Health Services program, focusing on a number of commonalities in several health-related occupations. Historical, ethical, and legal aspects are included along with the theoretical and practical aspects. The format is a combination of lecture, observation, and clinical experiences for allied health and nursing students.

The *case presentation model* is typically a problem-solving approach organized around practice situations that are common to a number of occupations. Using either real-life or simulated cases, this method is generally designed to initiate role sharing and information exchange and to facilitate the early stages of collaborative and interdependent teamwork. It does not require actual delivery of service or activity. Examples include the University of Minnesota program where the case study method is utilized to teach a combined class of students from nursing, medicine, and a number of allied health programs.

The *research team model* is a more intensive problem-solving approach, which is project- or product-oriented and generally focuses on a community need. An example might be a project in which students in different disciplines work together to produce a directory of community services.

The *patient care model* is generally found in a clinical setting where students participate in a collaborative, interdependent manner, focusing on the delivery of patient care, utilizing referral techniques, and learning to practice as a team. To date, most interdisciplinary efforts have utilized the patient care model, relying on the clinical education phase of occupational preparation to bring students together. For example, the Kentucky January project of the College of Allied Health Professions, University of Kentucky, places students from allied health programs in teams in rural communities, and another University of Kentucky project called SITE provides summer interdisciplinary team experience to students from medicine, dentistry, pharmacy, nursing, nutrition, physical therapy, physician assistant, and social work. Similarly, the Wayne State University extramural program assigns students from medicine, nursing, occupational therapy, pharmacy, physical therapy, and social work in teams to community service agencies. The State University of New York at Buffalo provides collaborative summer clinical experiences to students in physical therapy, occupational therapy, nursing, and rehabilitation counseling.

These four models of interdisciplinary education (common issue, case presentation, research, and patient care) can be carried out on a departmental project basis or by an institution-wide administrative unit. Connelly's (1978) review indicates that most interdisciplinary activity in allied health is carried out on a departmental project basis with outside funds. Consequently, the programs are often discontinued when initial start-up funds are exhausted.

According to Connelly, the project nature of most of the interdisciplinary activities in allied health has led to a labeling of these activities as "nonessential." This bias is strengthened by the fact that many interdisciplinary programs are conducted in summer sessions. Further, programs are often developed by project staff rather than faculty; thus these programs rarely become an integral part of disciplinary curricula.

The importance of faculty involvement for program development is dramatically demonstrated by a project underwritten by the W. K. Kellogg Foundation. As a recipient of a Kellogg Allied Health Instruction Personnel Grant, the University of California at San Francisco embarked on an ambitious project to develop objectives for a core curriculum and learning modules (Rosinski, 1977). From their experiences in formulating behavioral objectives, the project staff learned a painful lesson. Although the competencies reflected what numerous allied health administrators perceived to be essential, and the objectives, in turn, reflected the competencies, formulation of the objectives was almost solely the work of the project staff. Individuals who were to conduct a particular course at any one of the consortium institutions played little or no part in the formulation of objectives; consequently, many disagreed with them. What resulted was a set of thoroughly prepared objectives that, for many instructors, served no function. The original goal of having most of the curriculum embodied in learning modules was also abandoned because of the faculty's unwillingness to accept the formulated objectives. According to Connelly (1978, pp. 43-44):

> Interdisciplinary education seems to precipitate issues and problems both external and internal to the academic setting. Problems and concerns with administrative structures, faculty, and students are real internal issues for the interdisciplinary concept. With no single ownership, the interdisciplinary program appears to consume an inordinate amount of administrative and faculty time and resources. Students must deal with issues of adjusting their priorities and activities in order to involve themselves with interdisciplinary activities. Interdisciplinary programming requires an installation process in the academic unit that creates a need for change and unique approaches. Faculty and student incentive systems need to be reordered to adequately accommodate the interdisciplinary concept within the discipline oriented academic unit.
>
> External influences such as accreditation and professional politics are real factors in dealing with interdisciplinary activity. The continuation of separate discipline accreditation will not impede interdisciplinary activities but will definitely retard their proliferation. Professional objections to the interdisciplinary concept will only be overcome

> through demonstration of effectiveness in practice or pressures from consumer and/or governmental agencies.

A major stumbling block that needs to be overcome is the reluctance on the part of many allied health groups to participate in collaborative efforts. In a survey of 675 allied health, medical, pharmacy, nursing, dentistry, and other academic units, it was found that, while apparently supportive of the need for teaching the professional role in health care, allied health educators were less interested than their colleagues in medicine, pharmacy, and nursing in teaching collaboration skills (Marion, 1978). Apparently, allied health educators place a low priority on the role of interdisciplinary education in meeting program objectives for students. Connelly (1978) suggests that the reasons for this low rating include confusion regarding the philosophy and objectives of the concept, professional turf guarding, realization that extraordinary resources are necessary to provide students with interdisciplinary experiences, lack of preparation of faculty, and a definite shortage of information on successful models within allied health education.

The Center for Interdisciplinary Education in Allied Health was founded in 1976 at the College of Allied Health Professions, University of Kentucky, to assist educational programs in the development and operation of interdisciplinary activities designed to foster a team approach to the delivery of health care. Among the center's functions are resource and information sharing, training workshops, conferences, and research projects in teaching-learning methodologies and evaluation of interdisciplinary education programs. It is hoped that this new center will meet the required informational needs and prove to be a catalytic agent for the increased acceptance and utilization of interdisciplinary education in allied health.

Identifying Common Course Content. Clearly, the objectives of interdisciplinary education can be more effectively attained if common course content is identified. The term *core* is used to refer to this common course content. However, some confusion has arisen because the segments of educational content to which the term has been applied have varied from an entire program to a cluster of courses to modules within courses. The word *core* derives from the Latin word for heart; this implies that core content is at the heart of educational content and that it "provides the foundation for related information that is generic to all health categories and the specific curriculum designed to give the student the necessary knowledge and skills in his prime area of interest. The skills and training needed to perform a specific job can then be built upon by incorporating specialty training and clinical practice" (Harmon and Quinones, 1974, p. 54). However, core more frequently is used simply to refer to any course content that can be used in the preparation of more than one occupation. Even more confusing is the use of the term *core program* to refer to programs that use common course content in some way.

Confusion also arises from the fact that the terms *core curriculum* and *interdisciplinary education* have been used interchangeably. Interdisciplinary education refers to the educational process, whereas core curriculum refers to a set of educational materials common to more than one discipline or occupation. As previously noted, interdisciplinary education does not necessarily require core material, and core material is not necessarily used in an interdisciplinary context—although it should be developed through interdisciplinary collaboration.

The confusion surrounding this term should not obscure the potential value of identifying common areas of knowledge and skills that lend themselves to shared course content. Collegiate programs for allied health occupations generally embody three types of courses: (1) not specifically health related (part of the general education component discussed in Chapter Four); (2) health related but not specifically occupation related (might also be part of the general education component); and (3) occupation related (part of the occupational training component). The first two types of courses are more frequently shared than the third. A study of core curriculum projects by Burnett (1973) identified a variety of shared course areas, most of which were either not related to specific occupations or taught generic competencies such as counseling, teaching, administration, or research. These areas included:

- general education, especially English and mathematics
- biological and physical sciences, especially anatomy and physiology
- behavioral sciences, more prevalent among two-year college programs, usually including group counseling focused on interpersonal relations
- research, generally given in four-year programs, including some instruction in statistics and research methodology, and research experience
- teaching and learning methods, also generally given by four-year programs, including instruction in various methods to improve teacher effectiveness

In addition, programs sometimes share courses or portions of courses that teach general health-related knowledge, such as medical terminology, emergency procedures, human values, legal responsibilities, and ethics. For instance, the Commission on Interprofessional Education and Practice—which involves several colleges within the Ohio State University, the Columbus Cluster of Theological Schools, and a number of state chapters of professional associations—has developed core materials to train professional students and practicing professionals in emerging ethical issues. The commission offers interprofessional credit courses, including changing societal values and the professions, interprofessional care of the patient/client, and ethical issues common to the helping professions; it also offers continuing education programs and undertakes research projects. There are lessons to be learned from this commission in terms of bridging the gap between "the academic and practicing communities in identifying interprofessional issues and developing cooperative approaches to their solution" (Center for Interdisciplinary Education in Allied Health, 1979, p. 2).

In general, collaboration within disciplines to develop common course content has been hampered by the slow development of methodologies to identify and delineate tasks and functions performed within each occupational role. Professional associations, encouraged by federal support, are beginning to show greater interest in task analyses and role delineation studies. In response to the commission survey in 1978, 44 percent of the seventy-nine professional association respondents reported that they were actively involved in such studies; only 15 percent reported no such involvement.

Since the mid seventies, the federal government (Division of Associated Health Professions, Health Resources Administration) has supported a program of systematic role delineation studies for personnel in occupational therapy, respiratory therapy, radiologic technology, medical records, environmental health, and physician assistants. Most of these projects have been conducted by the professional associations themselves, with advice and guidance from educators, practitioners, related health professionals, and others. Consensus is reached—in some cases by task analyses and in others by groups of experts—on the entire range of tasks performed on the job, as well as on the minimal knowledge, skills, and behaviors required for successful performance. If different levels of personnel are involved, these required competencies are identified for the different levels. The delineations, then, are validated by studies of actual job performance. One of the major goals of the projects has been the design of curriculum guides, based on the roles and functions identified, which can be used by faculty in designing courses geared to achievement of the behavioral objectives. Although past projects may have been too dissimilar in methodology and content to use for the purpose of determining commonalities, collaboration in future projects could lead to the discovery of common grounds for sharing educational experiences. Identification of overlap in knowledge and skill requirements also would be useful in designing curricula for practitioners who can perform the multiple functions needed in certain practice settings.

Health Career Core and Technician-Level Generalist. In 1973, Kinsinger argued for a "health career core" for preparing health technician generalists. The core content would contain a broad background in both acute care and health maintenance and would include solid grounding in health care fundamentals. The training would prepare personnel to meet multiple manpower needs, particularly in medically underserved areas, reduce the overspecialization and proliferation of mid-level occupations, and provide students with wider career options and opportunities for mobility. It appears also that the costs of such a program would be lower than the accumulated costs of programs for practitioners whose functions are specialized (Kinsinger, 1973).

The outlook for health services and changing health manpower utilization patterns discussed in Chapter Three point to an increasing need for personnel who can function in a variety of settings and exercise a wide range of skills. Moreover, the fact that the functions of many allied health personnel, indeed most health personnel, overlap to a significant extent makes the concept of a generalist both rational and feasible.

The armed forces have trained and utilized generalists for years. Now there is growing interest in preparing assistants or technicians with cross-occupational knowledge and skills in the civilian sector as well. Already a number of programs for "multiple competency" training have been developed in response to local manpower needs, particularly in rural areas where economic considerations require efficient utilization of personnel. For example, the multiple competency clinical technicians program at the School of Community and Allied Health, University of Alabama, prepares students to combine roles and functions in medical assisting, x-ray, and medical laboratory work. A major experimental project in Southern Illinois University prepared students to perform in more than one occupational role in rural settings (Lugenbeel, 1979). These and similar projects have met with varying degrees of success, and many problems and questions still need to be addressed. Most critical are questions relating to selection of competency combinations, maintenance of high quality education without excessive lengthening of preparation, and appropriate credentialing mechanisms. Moreover, the support of professional associations has yet to be won in some instances.

A major task for the allied health professions and education in the coming decade will be to achieve some self-regulation congruent with the ideas of cost containment and accountability, with a strengthened public health and patient focus. A willingness to collaborate in education is a starting point. To continue with the proliferation of subspecialty after subspecialty will only serve to invite external regulation and increase public skepticism with regard to the motives of groups in the health fields.

Promises and Problems of Collaborative Efforts

Collaborative arrangements between institutions hold great promise for attaining a variety of objectives relating to cost, quality, accessibility, and continuity in allied health education. Today cost accountability has become a major concern of both educators and planners. The actual cost savings of collaborative activities in allied health education are difficult to measure. Clearly, costs are saved when program components are not unnecessarily duplicated or when resources are shared. However, collaborative activities are usually not designed to reduce services but rather to add services; consequently, they may lead to greater expenses. If new service needs can be met or the quality of educational processes can be raised at relatively low cost through collaboration, then the collaboration is cost-beneficial. Probably the most direct cost-saving approaches are those that involve agreements not to start programs at all (student exchanges) and those that lead to the establishment of temporary programs.

Although sharing of resources does not guarantee the quality of education, the potential for higher quality is enhanced with access to the facilities of a large university or medical center, and through the interaction and cooperation of various faculties. A further benefit of interinstitutional collaboration is seen in improved access, both in terms of students' access to programs and the public's access to health services. Many collaborative arrangements have been designed specifically to supply the necessary manpower for remote areas. The results reported by some of these programs indicate that although out-migration does occur, many graduates are remaining in their home communities to practice.

A potential benefit of collaboration that has only recently begun to be appreciated is continuity in learning. By planning together, educational institutions of different types preparing students for different levels of practice can remove some of the administrative barriers to a smooth transition from one learning environment to another. Establishing mechanisms that promote greater continuity between all aspects of learning benefits all society, not just students. Continuity makes education more efficient (and thus less costly) and, theoretically, more effective, by ensuring that the proper foundations for further learning are laid. To achieve broad-scale continuity in allied health education—between levels, disciplines, and educational components—will require collaboration not only between individual institutions but also among the various broad interest groups concerned with education and quality assurance.

Collaborative arrangements, for all their promise, are not always successful in achieving their goals. Many of the problems of collaboration are hardly specific to allied health but rather seem to be endemic to academia. Collaboration requires commitment, resources, negotiation and compromise, and a willingness to subordinate one's specific interest to a larger objective. Problems of collaboration also arise in instances of perceived status differences. Some four-year institutions are skeptical regarding the level of preparation in two-year colleges. This problem may be particularly acute in the case of allied health programs on university campuses where they are often outside the mainstream of campus life and, at times, struggling for academic recognition.

Movement toward a genuine alliance among health professionals must begin with educational programs and settings utilizing the commonalities in functions and knowledge bases of the various health occupations. The independent schools of allied health—discussed in Chapter Four—were developed largely to provide just such an educational setting. One important reason why these schools have not as yet completely fulfilled their potential in promoting shared learning experiences is that much of the curriculum planning is developed without the benefit of a systematic analysis and objective evaluation. This situation is being remedied in part by role delineation studies which, by carefully specifying functions of single occupations, provide a solid basis for determining shared educational content. Active involvement and support of professional associations, with input from educators, in conducting research on functional commonalities will be the key to recognition of similarities in knowledge and skill requirements on which to establish shared learning experiences. The problem of territorialism or turfdom cited earlier cannot be resolved without professional commitment to collaboration in education as well as practice. Similarly, the development of common course content depends on the active involvement and support of faculty in the various disciplines concerned. A further requirement of successful collaborative efforts would be to strengthen lines of communication among the various professional associations and between the professional associations and educators.

The outlook for increased collaboration within allied health education and between allied health and other health education is, on balance, favorable. There are forces inherent in allied health that make greater collaboration both necessary and possible. Factors known to have a positive influence on successful collaboration—diversity and complementarity of institutional resources, student body, and goals—characterize allied health to a greater degree than most other fields. In addition, collaborative efforts in allied health tend to be targeted toward specific rather than general purposes, thus facilitating clear understanding of roles, contributions, and objectives. The accreditation and credentialing processes, by setting certain basic standards for educational content in allied health, also may promote clarity in collaborative arrangements.

More general trends currently under way in postsecondary education can be expected to have some ameliorating effects on the obstacles to collaboration, particularly with respect to issues of articulation and continuity in learning. In the past decade, there evolved a new view of education as lifelong learning rather than a lock-stepped process with a well-defined beginning and end:

> Full opportunity to learn cannot be limited to the young; it must be for everyone, in any walk

> of life, for whatever purposes are beneficial. It cannot be reserved to a single period of life, it must be a recurrent opportunity: an opportunity to update a skill, to broaden the possibilities of a career whether old or new, or to add intellectual zest and cultural enrichment throughout life. No longer can it be the single opportunity of a lifetime; now it must become the total opportunity for a lifetime (Commission on Non-Traditional Study, 1973, p. 12).

Coupled with major changes in higher education attendance patterns—a decline in the growth rate for enrollments of the traditional college-age population and an increase in the number of adult learners—this new view of learning has brought about revisions in educational policies and procedures facilitating the entry and progress of nontraditional students, has increased tolerance for "stepping out" (leaving and reentering the study process) and for students transferring from other institutions, and has accelerated interest in proficiency and equivalency exams and evaluation of experiential learning. The rapid growth of extension and continuing education centers as well as of nontraditional forms of study attests to the growing emphasis on lifelong learning. These changes, by gradually shifting the focus from formal educational credentials to performance-based competencies, will surely have positive consequences for greater continuity between learning experiences in allied health education. Finally, postsecondary education has become highly sensitive to the pressures for accountability and cost-effectiveness. Rather than be subject to external regulation, the general preference is toward voluntary collaborative arrangements both between and within institutions. As these arrangements become more prevalent, the pressure on allied health educators to produce their own special solutions should be reduced.

VI

Future Directions: Commission Recommendations and Steps to Achieve Them

The recommendations set forth in this chapter are the consensus of the commission on the future directions that allied health education should take to improve its quality, accessibility, continuity, and cost-effectiveness. As previously stated, not all these recommendations represent new ideas, nor are all of them action oriented. Some have been offered elsewhere but have not been readily accepted or implemented. They are emphasized here again as guiding principles for educational planning because the commission believes that adherence to them will improve the quality and efficiency of both education and health care. Further, experimentation in allied health occupations and education over the past decade has yielded methodologies that can help implement goals that were once only theoretical ideals. Some recommendations calling for action are novel; others that have been tried before and proven successful are offered in the belief that these earlier efforts should now be implemented on a wider scale and modified as necessary to accommodate local needs and conditions, changed realities, or larger audiences.

These recommendations reflect six basic themes discussed and agreed upon by the commissioners:

1. Allied health personnel provide essential health care services, and these services will become increasingly important in the future for achieving national health goals.

2. Allied health education is essential for provision of a competent and sufficient health workforce. Allied health education should be viewed as a continuous, rather than discrete, process which has four components: basic occupational preparation, job education and training, advanced education, and continuing education. The minimum competencies to enter any allied health occupation may be acquired in many ways. However, the level of knowledge and skills needed for most allied health occupations is such that formal postsecondary education is the best assurance that a sufficient number of competent practitioners are prepared. Settings for formal basic occupational preparation include collegiate institutions, hospitals and other health care providers, postsecondary noncollegiate institutions, and the armed forces. The basic preparation may range, depending on practice level, from short-term preparation through doctoral studies. In addition, formal postsecondary education—not necessarily in collegiate institutions—is the most favorable environment for updating competencies and for developing leadership capabilities, which are essential for meeting changing health service needs. This theme represents a departure from the emphasis of the 1967 subcommittee on collegiate settings. The commission believes that there is insufficient evidence to recommend one type of setting over another; moreover, the current diversity of allied health education settings reflects the great diversity among allied health services. (See Chapter Four for a description of the various types of settings with formal allied health programs; all of these settings are referred to here as educational institutions.)

3. The primary purpose of allied health education is to

prepare students for health service; therefore, it is clear that educational processes must be related to practice needs and viewed as a means of achieving standard performance objectives. Role delineation projects offer the best available means for linking education more closely to practice needs. Further, the right to practice should be based on achievement of these performance objectives rather than on receipt of an academic degree. The educational institution—collegiate or noncollegiate—has the responsibility of preparing students to meet these objectives.

4. Because of the dynamic nature of health service delivery, flexibility in the educational processes for preparing students to meet these performance objectives is essential for promoting growth, innovation, and progress. A monolithic approach to allied health education is unrealistic and would result in stagnation.

5. The educational processes for health occupations should place the interests of the student or the public to be served above any special interest of educational institutions and professional groups. Whenever there is any conflict, it should be resolved in favor of the student or the public.

6. To avoid duplication and waste, coordination of resources and collaborative problem solving are essential. Whenever possible, the following four steps are encouraged: demonstration projects, evaluation and assessment of successful methodologies, dissemination, and implementation on a wider scale of successful projects. Continuity in funding to support all four steps is crucial for successful implementation of these recommendations.

The commission recommendations address issues and problems in six major areas: (1) strengthening alliances in service and education, (2) determining appropriate content and level of educational programs, (3) improving clinical education, (4) building the capability for leadership and innovation, (5) providing for planning and administration without waste, and (6) supplying adequate funding. Fifteen of the recommendations are considered by the commission to be primary and of equal importance in solving these problems. The commission also offers sixty-three corollaries to implement the objectives of its primary recommendations, but it recognizes that there are other ways of meeting these goals that may be just as effective. (Note that the primary recommendations are numbered consecutively; corollaries are double-numbered.) The fifteen primary recommendations are as follows:

1. *Alliance in service and education should be strengthened, based on an appreciation of the interdependence of all health occupations and an understanding of their roles, functions, and special contributions.*
2. *Education should be linked to practice through role delineations.*
3. *Allied health education should prepare students who can meet standard performance objectives and adapt to changing health service needs; flexibility in the methods of preparation should be encouraged.*
4. *To meet new service demands, all allied health educational programs should include the study of (a) human values, (b) illness prevention and health promotion methods, and (c) delivery systems, including roles and functions of health personnel, patients' rights, legal risks, cost-effectiveness, and quality control.*
5. *In the future, new health service needs should be met, where possible, without establishing new occupations and programs; unnecessary expansion of entry-level requirements should be controlled.*
6. *The importance of continuing education should be recognized and networks should be established to ensure collaboration and information sharing on continuing education matters.*
7. *Clinical and didactic education should be better integrated; and the range and types of clinical education sites and methods should be expanded to meet new health service demands.*
8. *Research in clinical education methods and theory must be greatly expanded.*
9. *The development of leadership in the clinical, managerial, and educational areas should be a priority for allied health education.*
10. *Support for research on allied health education should be*

substantially increased, and allied health faculty should be encouraged to strengthen their commitment to research.

11. *Educational institutions should strengthen their efforts to increase the representation of minorities and women in leadership positions.*
12. *The establishment, expansion, maintenance, reduction, and termination of allied health programs should be based on manpower requirements, adequacy and efficient use of available resources, and collaboration within and among educational and other institutions.*
13. *Educational and collaborating institutions should adopt mechanisms to facilitate the removal of unnecessary barriers to student progress.*
14. *Information relating to administration and planning in allied health education should be collected and shared systematically.*
15. *Significantly increased funding for allied health should be provided at the federal, state, and local government levels and from private resources.*

Strengthening Alliances in Service and Education

Recommendation 1: *Alliance in service and education should be strengthened, based on an appreciation of the interdependence of all health occupations and an understanding of their roles, functions, and special contributions.*

The past decade has been characterized by growth and affluence but also by discord among the many interest groups in allied health. The period of austerity now facing all health services and education presents many challenges for health occupations but may yield hidden benefits as well by forcing greater commitment to innovation and to formation of new alliances among those involved.

After years of growth pains and identity struggles, the commission detects a new spirit of cooperation in the field. There seems to be a greater willingness, at least on the part of some allied health occupations, to work with each other and with other health occupations. This new spirit should be fostered by providing adequate information regarding the roles, functions, and contributions of each health occupation and by promoting a better appreciation of the interdependence of all health services. Alliances need to be built and strengthened between education and service, between allied health and other occupations, and within allied health services and education. The answer to the problems of the next decade lies in communication, cooperation, collaboration, and sharing of resources. It is significant that the new emblem chosen this year for the Allied Health Education Newsletter, published by the Department of Allied Health Evaluation of the American Medical Association, reads: coordination, cooperation, collaboration. This theme is repeated by many of the professional associations responding to the commission survey and clearly points the way for the future. Further, the ultimate impact of the commission recommendations depends on the creation and nurture of these new alliances.

Determining Appropriate Content and Level of Educational Programs

Education for health occupations is a resource for persons within the community, state, and nation. Therefore, the educational process for health occupations should be addressed to the needs of consumers—including students, as consumers of the education, and the public at large, as consumers of the services the graduates will provide.

In the opinion of this commission, the needs of consumers are best served when allied health education is accomplished in the most efficient and cost-effective manner, with emphasis on preparing students to meet health service demands. Although allied health education should be related to performance objectives based on these demands, this does not require that it be limited to technical skill preparation. Students will need an adequate knowledge base to permit adjustment throughout their working years to a rapidly changing health care delivery system. The importance of knowledge preparation relative to skill preparation increases with each higher level of education. Moreover, the educational program should help students to understand and relate to the human as well as physical needs of patients and clients.

The commission recommendations in this section are directed at achieving these major goals related to appropriate content and level of programs in allied health education:

- linking education to practice
- assuring flexibility
- meeting new health service demands
- slowing down the proliferation of occupations and programs
- recognizing the continuum of education

Recommendation 2: *Education should be linked to practice through role delineations.*

Today a gap exists between declaration and attainment of the goal of relating education to performance objectives based on health service demands. Current knowledge of practice needs is limited for most allied health occupations. Consequently, educational content is determined by expert judgment and the tendency is to err in favor of too much rather than too little education.

Recognizing this knowledge gap, many professional associations are giving considerable attention to the identification of the roles and functions of the personnel they represent. In response to the commission survey of seventy-nine professional associations, 44 percent reported very active involvement in task analysis or role delineation studies, and only 15 percent reported no such involvement.

The federal government, through the Division of Associated Health Professions (DAHP) of the Bureau of Health Manpower, has supported the most comprehensive and systematic program of role delineation projects for physician assistants and personnel in occupational therapy, respiratory therapy, radiologic technology, medical records, and environmental health.

The projects have utilized advisory committees composed of experts from various sectors, including employers, practitioners, medical specialists who use the services of personnel in the occupation under study, educators, and representatives of government agencies.

A typical role delineation project should ideally include the following components, although not all of the professional associations involved have completed or implemented the total process:

1. *Delineation of roles and functions.* Consensus is reached—in some cases by task analyses and in others by groups of experts—on the range of tasks performed on the job and the minimum basic knowledge, skills, and behavior required for successful performance. If different levels of personnel are involved, the tasks are organized by competency levels. Roles and functions thus determined are then validated by studies of actual job performance.
2. *Development of curriculum guides/curriculum workshops.* Curriculum guides are developed on the basis of these job descriptions, and workshops are held to show faculty how to use these guides for designing courses geared to the achievement of behavioral objectives.
3. *Design of examinations.* Criterion-referenced examinations are designed to permit entry to practice through demonstration of competencies shown to be essential by role delineation study. Currently, most professional associations require completion of educational requirements in order to sit for these examinations. For a few occupations, such as physician assistant, a degree is not required and the right to practice is based solely on demonstration of competency.
4. *Design of self-assessment kits.* Discipline-oriented kits are designed, either for a whole field or a specific area, to allow the practitioner to identify and profile his or her own deficiencies. These kits are particularly useful for identifying continuing education needs and planning for individualized learning experiences.
5. *Continuous updating.* The entire process must be repeated

periodically to ensure currency, since practice patterns change constantly.

The role delineation process, when carried out fully in this manner, allows standardization of educational objectives by linking them closely to practice needs. It also provides a mechanism through which the continuous competence of the practitioner can be assured. Further, it is the first step in determining commonalities in practice and educational needs of various allied health occupations—a goal persistently heard throughout the last ten years. The potential of role delineation methodology is still untapped for laying the foundation for realistic sharing of educational experience. Results of role delineation studies can be used to develop a knowledge base generic to many allied health occupations, to plan more effectively for interdisciplinary education, and to implement cross-occupational (multicompetency) programs that are based on demonstrated commonalities in function. Role delineation study findings can also be utilized most effectively to meet new service demands without adding to the proliferation or duplication of programs and occupations.

The various role delineation projects supported by the DAHP over the past years have developed increasingly sophisticated methodologies and have provided valuable models for other groups. Sharing the lessons learned on these projects would save substantial time and costs for new projects and would encourage greater comparability of the results of these new projects. Unfortunately, lack of collaboration and communication among the different groups involved in role delineation studies in the past has resulted in products of value to particular occupations but not sufficiently comparable to serve as a basis for identifying commonalities.

2.1: *The federal government or a private foundation should provide adequate funding to an organization representing broad interests in allied health education (such as ASAHP) for a four-stage project to promote more effective use of role delineation studies.*

a. *"Lessons Learned Workshop" and Development of Manual.* The workshops should convene the staff of professional organizations and DAHP who have had primary responsibility for DAHP-funded role delineations projects in order to share methods, to identify problem areas, results, successes, and failures, and to explore new ideas, concepts, and solutions. The product of the workshop should be a procedure manual outlining the most efficient and effective methods for developing and validating role delineations, developing curriculum guides, designing evaluation and self-assessment instruments, and continuous updating. The manual should emphasize that role delineation study necessitates collaboration among many groups, including practitioners, employers, educators, and others.

b. *National meeting of allied health professional organizations on role delineation development, and establishment of study groups to determine commonalities in practice requirements.* A national meeting, led by participants in the Lessons Learned Workshop, should bring together broad representation from professional organizations to explain the use of the procedure manual. The meeting should also encourage the establishment of study groups to compare roles, functions, and competency requirements and identify those that are common to two or more occupations.

c. *Regional workshops to develop strategies for advocating and explaining the use of role delineations by faculty.* Regional workshops should be conducted in cooperation with other educational associations and regional coordinating bodies (for example, the Southern Regional Education Board) to develop strategies for more effective and widespread use of role delineations by faculty. Participants should be prepared to implement these strategies and should be encouraged to hold subsequent workshops within each state on methods of translating role delineations into curriculum.

d. *The results of these meetings and workshops should be widely disseminated by the coordinating organization.*

Recommendation 3: *Allied health education should prepare students who can meet standard performance objectives and adapt to changing health service needs; flexibility in the methods of preparation should be encouraged.*

The commission believes that allied health education programs should provide students with at least the minimum knowledge and skills needed to perform effectively in an occupational role in any geographic location or setting in the nation. These skills should be closely linked to practice needs and standardized through role delineation studies. However, the commission also believes that flexibility is essential both for practitioners and for educational processes.

In a rapidly changing health service delivery system, adaptability will be essential. The basic occupational preparation program should be viewed as a foundation for continued learning and development so that graduates do not find themselves with obsolete skills and without the background to develop new skills. A broad foundation, as opposed to restricted skill training, is particularly important in occupational areas that require lengthy preparation. Waste resulting from education that is not used is greater if the time invested in education is longer.

Adaptability and flexibility can be developed in several ways: (1) by acquiring a knowledge base generic to health occupations, on which the knowledge and skills of several specialties can be built; (2) by learning the competencies required to perform in more than one occupational role; and (3) by developing broadly based scientific and analytical capabilities through study in the arts and sciences.

Additional research by both professional groups and educators will be necessary to identify aspects of a knowledge base that are required both within and across clusters of health occupations. A starting point for these studies would be a comparison of roles and functions, as well as knowledge and skill requirements, of different occupations.

> 3.1: *Demonstration projects to design and implement curriculum modules based on role delineations for two or more occupations should be funded.* Projects should be conducted by faculty in collaboration with professional association study groups on commonalities (see Corollary 2.1). Each project should be evaluated and the procedures and results widely disseminated. Both two-year and four-year institutions with an appropriate program mix should be encouraged to apply for demonstration project funds. The federal government or a private foundation should subsequently fund implementation of the most promising approaches by other institutions.

The idea of preparing people for more than one occupational role is not new. It has been proposed, tried, and frequently has been met with strong resistance from professional groups. Several years ago, for example, the World Health Organization issued a position paper recommending multicompetency education for rehabilitation personnel in developing countries; the proposal was greeted with dismay. Attempts in Canada to prepare occupational and physical therapists in a single program also failed, primarily because of lack of support from professional groups.

Recently, however, interest in the idea has been renewed, as evidence is beginning to build that persons who can perform functions in more than one occupational category are valuable to employers in small rural hospitals or clinics and in some of the growing health delivery settings such as industry, where such flexibility is needed (see Chapter Three). Several educational institutions have already developed programs to prepare personnel for cross-occupational roles. Further, the armed forces have traditionally prepared health personnel for both a primary and secondary occupation. The lessons learned from these experiences should be shared with others interested in establishing similar programs.

> 3.2: *ASAHP should conduct a workshop for directors of allied health programs preparing students for more than one occupational role to identify similarities and differences in educational objectives, content, and procedures of these programs.* Representatives of relevant professional associations should also be involved in this workshop. The results of the workshop should be widely disseminated.

Studies of humanities, social sciences, and natural sciences can help allied health students acquire values, knowledge, and intellectual skills of great relevance for competent and humanistic practice as health care specialists, and they provide the broad-based scientific and analytical capabilities to build a foundation for further growth and adaptability. In its survey of leaders, the commission asked: "How important is each of the following areas of study in preparing for a career like yours?" Over half the academic and clinical leaders endorsed arts and humanities as very important, four fifths of academic leaders and three fifths of clinical leaders endorsed social sciences as very important, and about three fourths of leaders in each group endorsed basic biological sciences as very important.

In *programs below the baccalaureate or equivalent level,* study in the humanities, social sciences, and natural sciences should be included to reflect current health service needs and the demands of the employer. *Baccalaureate, master's, or equivalent programs* should provide more latitude in the inclusion of elements in these areas, based on current and future health service needs and on the value of the subject matter for preparing adaptable personnel who can relate to new technologies and a broad range of problems, situations, and settings. All doctoral programs should include elements in these areas that develop the capability to generate new knowledge and provide historical perspective on health service.

3.3: *Students in collegiate allied health education programs should be allowed significant opportunities for selection of courses in humanities, social sciences, and natural sciences, in keeping with the students' individual talents and interests for personal enrichment.*

In order to make the best use of existing resources and to ensure that students receive academic credit for these courses, allied health programs should arrange wherever possible for students to participate in general university courses. This point is reiterated in Corollary 13.7. In order to assure the relevancy of the subject matter, closer links should be developed between arts and sciences and allied health faculty.

3.4: *Allied health programs should develop mechanisms to permit allied health faculty to hold joint appointments and remain active in those disciplines in which they have completed graduate study.*

3.5: *Particularly at the graduate level, academic departments of allied health should provide appointments for faculty whose preparation is in the sciences or humanities and who may not be qualified as allied health practitioners.* These appointments should carry with them opportunities to participate fully in overall program planning.

Flexibility in allied health educational processes is necessary to permit innovation and creativity and to avoid stagnation. Flexibility is needed also to permit programs to build additional knowledge and skills that meet particular local health service needs. Market studies with local employers may identify needs that are not being met by programs addressed only to minimum national standards. In particular, flexibility is needed for programs preparing personnel to perform functions in more than one occupational role, because different combinations of cross-occupational knowledge and skills may be useful in different settings and geographical locations.

The accreditation mechanisms, which currently are undergoing close scrutiny, should assure flexibility as well as quality. Separate accreditation for each specialty limits flexibility. Moreover, when new specialties or combinations of specialties develop, educators and professional associations should evaluate experimental programs preparing people for these specialties before developing quality assurance mechanisms. Any eventual quality assurance mechanisms for personnel with cross-occupational knowledge and skills should not freeze particular combinations or approaches but should encourage those that meet local needs while assuring that the graduate's knowledge and skills in at least one occupational area are transferable to other geographic locations.

The National Commission on Allied Health Education (NCAHE) commends the Council on Postsecondary Accreditation (COPA) on its efforts to deal effectively with the proliferation of accrediting activities in the health care areas. The NCAHE agrees with the position stated by COPA: "It is not practical or desirable that *every* specialization be subject to *all* forms of quality assurances. Licensure or certification may be sufficient in the areas where society requires some sort of indication as to minimum professional competence; accreditation of an educational program does not serve to assure the specific qualifications of an individual." The COPA statement further indicates that "for educational activities where there is no compelling social need for licensure, certification, or accreditation, there are other useful ways to promote and improve quality through existing associations" (Task Force on Proliferation, 1977, p. 2). Again, the NCAHE concurs in this position.

> **Recommendation 4:** *To meet new service demands, all allied health educational programs should include the study of (a) human values, (b) illness prevention and health promotion methods, and (c) delivery systems, including roles and functions of health personnel, patients' rights, legal risks, cost-effectiveness, and quality control.*

Trends in health service and changing health priorities indicate the need to include the following subject areas which are health related but not occupationally specific and which currently are not a standard part of most allied health curricula: human values, prevention of illness and promotion of health, and delivery systems, including an appreciation of the roles and responsibilities of each health occupation, patients' rights, and legal risks. These topics lend themselves particularly well to interdisciplinary study.

Although the technological advances, growth, and specialization in health care delivery have led to great improvements in the treatment of disease and disability, they have also resulted in the impersonalization of health services. Consumers are becoming increasingly vocal in demanding more personal care and greater consideration for their needs as human beings. The increase in age and heterogeneity of the population of the United States has intensified the need for sensitivity in providing health services to the elderly and the handicapped and to persons of different ethnic groups.

The most effective means of communicating sensitivity toward patients is through teacher and practitioner role models. (The need to develop strong role models is addressed in recommendations on leadership development.) In addition, during the past decade, there has been increasing attention to the need to introduce instruction in human values into the curriculum for health personnel. Ronald W. McNeur of the Society for Health and Human Values estimates that approximately 100 of the 150 medical schools now offer instruction in human values. Topics related to human values are covered in separate courses, woven throughout the curriculum, included in clinical practicum, and/or taught as continuing education. Some allied health units also have developed and used courses and course modules in human values, with particular emphasis on gerontology (for example, the College of Community and Allied Health Professions at the University of Tennessee, the School of Allied Health at the University of Connecticut, the School of Allied Health at the State University of New York at Stonybrook, and

Erie Community College). Moreover, educators are beginning to recognize that a study of human values topics benefits even those in occupations with no direct patient contact (for example, cytotechnology) by helping those personnel recognize the impact of services they provide on human lives.

The commission believes that all health personnel should have at least a minimum appreciation of the impact of illness on the patient and the patient's family. Practitioners with patient contact should also have an understanding of cultural values and attitudes about illness and health care of ethnic groups in the community they serve.

Similarly, disease prevention has become a national priority because of growing recognition of its potential impact on improving the quality of life and reducing health expenditures. Allied health personnel in their various occupational roles can contribute to the prevention of disease and disability by helping patients and the public develop more healthy life styles and/or by effecting changes in the environment. The preventive approach to health service involves a major change in orientation from acute care to continuous care and a new emphasis on maintaining health. Corresponding shifts in the orientation and emphasis of allied health education will be necessary to prepare students for the new approach to practice. With the exception of a few occupational programs (for example, health education), the emphasis of allied health education in the United States today tends to be on human biology and health care organization rather than environment and life-style. Students in allied health programs associated with public health or in schools that combine public and allied health orientation are more likely than others to receive some exposure to prevention, but even for such students the exposure is likely to be fragmentary and without an established focus on health.

The commission supports the recommendation of the 1975 conference of health educators and health planning leaders convened by the Bureau of Health Education (Center for Disease Control) which states: "Education resources preparing students for careers in health administration, teaching, community development, and social work, as well as the medical, health, and allied health professions, shall be encouraged to require at least one course in (health) educational concepts and methodologies; continuing education and training courses in this subject shall also be encouraged" (Ogden, 1977, p. 150). Students in allied health programs should have an understanding of the thesis that disease and disability may occur as a result of interaction with the environment. They should become familiar with the appraisal of health hazards and the influence of personal characteristics.

Educational programs should prepare students to enter the work environment with some sense of their roles and responsibilities in relation to other health personnel, patients, and the employer. An effective health alliance can be forged if there is a mutual understanding of the importance of the services provided by various categories of health personnel and the roles and functions of each, including the range and limits of independent action they may be expected to take. Because of the diversity of health occupations and services, the need for a formal orientation on the topic is great.

Students should also receive preparation in legal risk management—particularly patients' rights and practitioners' responsibilities toward the patient. Another area of responsibility that deserves attention in the curriculum is cost and quality control. All of these topics relating to roles and responsibilities are almost universally neglected in allied health education today. Depending on educational level, the processes of these studies may range from short modules to entire courses. However, care should be taken not to lengthen the program unnecessarily. Further, interdisciplinary study of these topics is strongly encouraged.

New instructional materials are needed in these three broad subject areas of human values, illness prevention and health promotion, and delivery systems. Not all educational programs will have the resources to develop these new materials independently; moreover, it would not be cost-effective for each program to duplicate the efforts of others.

4.1: *The federal government and/or private foundations should support projects to develop interdisciplinary instructional modules in human values, prevention, and management and coordination of services, and to introduce the modules in the curriculum of educational programs.* Successful modules should be made widely available to educational institutions and also to employers and professional groups for in-service training and continuing education. The federal government should subsequently fund implementation of the most promising approaches by a limited number of other institutions. Special attention should be given to the needs of two-year colleges, private career schools, hospitals, and other educational institutions for modules to prepare technicians, assistants, and aides in these subject areas without undue lengthening of the total preparation time.

4.2: *Faculty development workshops and continuing education courses should be designed specifically to prepare faculty to integrate these topics in the courses they teach and/or in clinical instruction.*

Recommendation 5: *In the future, new health service needs should be met, where possible, without establishing new occupations and programs; unnecessary expansion of entry-level requirements should be controlled.*

Kinsinger (1973, p. 12) has noted that "the frantic scramble to develop 'new careers' in the health field has become an unending exercise" and that "in a time of unlimited affluence and plentiful educational resources this might have had some validity, but such planning is developing a manpower overhead that may soon collapse under its own weight." Unnecessary proliferation of basic occupational programs for new health specialties is wasteful and results in increased splintering of health service functions, which impairs the quality and increases the costs of health service delivery. However, the current tendency to create new occupations to meet each newly identified health service need will continue unless there is concerted effort on the part of educators, professional associations, accreditation bodies, and planners to seek alternative ways of meeting these needs.

What are some of the alternatives? In some cases, new health service needs can be met by providing supplemental preparation to existing health personnel or incorporating new objectives in existing educational programs rather than establishing separate programs for new specialties. For example, after a clinical health education program fell victim to retrenchment at the State University of New York at Stonybrook, it resurfaced in a different form—not as a formal major, but as a new component of other ongoing programs. The experience demonstrated that the preparation could be incorporated in existing programs and that a separate occupational preparation program was not needed.

In some cases, new health needs can be met by providing supplemental preparation to persons with general education backgrounds. Many health services require a foundation of knowledge in nonhealth disciplines plus short-term preparation in specific health applications—for example, services relating to special problems in the areas of mental health, social health, and health promotion. On the basis of the deliberations of the Advisory Panel on Health Service Needs, the commission believes that there will be increased attention in the coming years to health promotion, to the needs of the elderly and the handicapped, and to such problems as alcoholism, drug abuse, and smoking. If history were to repeat itself, it is likely that colleges and universities would start new basic occupational programs for new titles, such as "smoking cessation therapist," to meet newly emphasized health needs, whereas short-term preparation of college graduates who are seeking marketable skills would be more efficient.

Moreover, it may be appropriate for certain health services to be delivered by persons such as teachers or staff in social service agencies who have contact with client populations in nonhealth roles. Good examples of this alternative are the short programs in which thousands of fire fighters and police officers have been trained for emergency medical care.

5.1: *Funds should be provided for projects demonstrating ways of meeting new health service needs without creating new occupations or specialties, such as:*

- short-term supplemental preparation for existing health personnel
- short-term preparation in health applications for college graduates who majored in relevant nonhealth fields, such as psychology, sociology, and education—such programs should be developed in consultation with educators from these nonhealth fields
- in-service training programs for persons employed in nonhealth occupations who have contact with the patient/client population
- incorporation of new objectives in existing programs

The health service needs addressed in these demonstration projects should be identified in cooperation with local employers, agencies, and/or health planning groups. The federal government or a private foundation should subsequently fund implementation of the most promising approaches by a limited number of other institutions. In addition, allied health educators and professional groups are encouraged to work together to examine the feasibility of preparing generalists or persons with cross-occupational competencies.

One of the most significant trends in allied health education over the past decade, along with the splintering of occupations and specialties, has been the continuous expansion of educational requirements for entry into practice. In some cases, this expansion has involved a lengthening of time or contact hours required for degree completion. In others, it has involved the establishment of a higher degree level as the standard for employment. Arguments in favor of expanding educational requirements center on quality issues, the critical nature of the services provided, and the ever-increasing knowledge base. However, pressures for accountability to students and cost containment require that the greater student and public investment in learning be justified on the basis of practice needs.

Generally, there are few pressures on institutions to justify lengthened educational programs on the basis of practice needs. An exception is the action taken by the Texas Coordinating Board (1978) in response to requests for baccalaureate programs in nuclear medicine technology. The board surveyed technologists employed in this occupation and found that the vast majority had an associate degree or certificate; among the few prepared in a bachelor's program, most felt that the higher level of preparation was unnecessary, and some even reported that on-the-job training would have been adequate. The commission believes that educational administrators have the responsibility to make better use of role delineation studies in the future and/or follow-up studies of graduates and their employers to assure that the level and length of each program is appropriate.

Educational institutions, however, are not alone responsible for the education inflation in allied health. They are influenced by strong motivating forces to lengthen educational programs. One such force is state formula funding policies based on full-time equivalent enrollments. These policies, which encourage institutions to enroll students for as long as possible, run counter to cost containment considerations. Besides promoting a lengthening of standard programs, they discourage institutions from trying nontraditional approaches, such as flexible scheduling and the use of equivalency examinations, which might shorten the contact hours for some students. The commission has recommended in a subsequent section that states with formula funding policies based on full-time equivalent enrollments should reexamine these policies because the incentive for lengthening contact hours has a negative impact on cost containment and innovation.

In addition, accreditation standards have had an impact in some cases through an upgrading of the minimum degree requirements. Pressures for such upgrading from the professional associations result largely from perceptions of greater rewards attached to higher degrees. Only occasionally is serious consideration given to the relation of the educational requirements to practice needs, as identified in role delineation studies. A recent example is the revision of standards for respiratory therapy personnel based on role delineation studies conducted by the

American Association for Respiratory Therapy, discussed in Chapter Four. The use of role delineation studies in this instance put an end to unjustified inflation of entry-level preparation for respiratory therapists, while opening the possibility of preparing higher-level personnel for advanced functions. In other instances, role delineations might demonstrate that lengthened entry-level preparation is, in fact, justified.

> 5.2: *Public support for and accreditation of allied health programs should be linked to justification of the level and length of programs based on competencies needed and utilized in the delivery of health service.* This is particularly important when: (a) different degrees are being offered for the same occupational preparation; (b) a proposal is made that the entry-level requirement be raised; (c) a proposal is made for preparing a new specialty or level.

The influence of accreditation and the influence of certification go hand in hand. Although the educational institution has the responsibility to prepare competent practitioners, the right to practice should ideally be determined by demonstration of competency rather than degree. However, many certifying bodies have contributed to the inflation of educational credentials by using educational attainment and completion of approved programs as an indicator of preparedness for practice. In part, this reliance on educational criteria rather than demonstrated competency has been necessitated by the lamentable gap in information on practice needs and the questionable validity of testing mechanisms. The National Commission for Health Certifying Agencies (NCHCA), an umbrella organization of professional associations and credentialing bodies, has taken the leadership in moving toward more widespread development of standards and procedures to permit assessment of occupational preparation on the basis of professional/technical knowledge and skills rather than on the basis of overall program length and/or academic degree awarded. To meet this objective, NCHCA has set as a criterion for membership in Category A (the category restricted to certifying agencies) the provision of alternative routes to eligibility for certification other than formal education. This criterion will be in force by 1982. This commission agrees with the NCHCA that the right to practice should be based on competency and makes two additional recommendations for achieving this objective:

5.3: *The National Commission for Health Certifying Agencies should adopt, as a criterion for accepting certifying agencies as members, that certification and recertification mechanisms must be based on validated role delineations.* This criterion should be in force no later than 1985.

5.4: *Funds should be provided for research to improve the methodology of performance-based testing.*

Recommendation 6: *The importance of continuing education should be recognized and networks should be established to ensure collaboration and information sharing on continuing education matters.*

Greater emphasis should be placed on the learning continuum and the role of continuing and advanced education to meet expanding subspecialty needs or personal enrichment goals without expanding the content or length of preparation for entry-level employment in an occupation. As stated earlier, in a rapidly changing health care delivery system, with new technological advances to be expected over the coming years, it is appropriate to envision basic occupational preparation not as the sole source of the entire body of knowledge in a discipline but as a foundation for further learning.

The commission's survey of professional associations revealed that continuing education is one of their major areas of concern. A full 97 percent of the seventy-nine responding associations were involved in assessing continuing education needs, 82 percent in offering continuing education courses, 81 percent in setting and/or reviewing continuing education standards, and

76 percent in designing continuing education curriculum guidelines or materials.

The Conference on Continuing Education sponsored by ASAHP in 1978 provided a forum for educators, professional association representatives, practitioners, providers, and other interested groups to discuss and attempt to resolve together the major issues in continuing education, including mandatory versus voluntary continuing education, accreditation, credit, curriculum approval, needs assessment, delivery systems, financing, records, and utilization. The momentum from this conference should not be lost. There is a need for a permanent forum for collective problem solving on continuing education matters and collective development of guidelines for ensuring the quality and relevancy to practice of course offerings. An umbrella organization, such as ASAHP, which brings together the many interest groups concerned about continuing allied health education, could provide this forum for problem solving as well as offer essential information and research services. Although there is evidence of an explosion of continuing education activities, information on these activities has never been compiled systematically and in a way that would facilitate cross-occupational exchanges. One reason for lack of a systematic ongoing effort to facilitate communication and exchange of continuing education matters is that such activities are not covered by any health-related federal funding program. Information on continuing education programs should be collated by topic area, and interdisciplinary program networks should be encouraged, particularly at the regional and local levels. Dissemination of research on continuing education and new research in areas of broad concern also are needed.

> 6.1: *A National Coalition for Continuing Education should be established to provide leadership and services at national, regional, and local levels.* This voluntary coalition is intended as a forum for collective problem solving, information sharing, and research; it should facilitate rather than regulate continuing education processes. The ongoing functions should include: (a) collective de-

velopment of guidelines and principles for continuing education activities; (b) support services and technical assistance for establishing and publicizing local and regional interdisciplinary continuing education networks; (c) clearinghouse for research on continuing education; and (d) consumer information services (for example, to members, practitioners). Participants in the coalition should be representatives of educational institutions, professional associations, practitioners, employers, and accrediting, certifying, and licensing bodies. Initial support should be provided by federal government or private sources to establish this coalition, which should become self-supporting. Once the ongoing services are in operation, the coalition could become a center for research in continuing education.

Improving Clinical Education

Many of the problems and challenges facing allied health education apply to clinical as well as didactic education. Both components should relate to practice needs, prepare competent and humane practitioners, and foster mutual appreciation and collaboration among the professions. Unnecessary duplication of required clinical practicum, like unnecessary duplication of coursework, is wasteful; therefore, the use of equivalency examinations and other methods of demonstrating competency already attained is encouraged.

The commission believes that interdisciplinary learning experiences are beneficial in promoting cooperation and collaboration in practice. In many ways, the clinical setting lends itself well to interdisciplinary education: Here, students and practitioners from various occupations with functional commonalities can be brought together to apply their complementary knowledge and skills to a health care problem. The commission encourages continued efforts to arrange clinical experiences that foster collaboration, such as that provided in the Kentucky January model.

The commission recommendations in this section are directed at achieving these major goals:

- assuring better integration of clinical and didactic education
- expanding the range of clinical education sites and methods
- strengthening research in clinical education methods and theory

The issue of preparation for clinical leadership is taken up in the subsequent section dealing with leadership development.

> **Recommendation 7:** *Clinical and didactic education should be better integrated; and the range and types of clinical education sites and methods should be expanded to meet new health service demands.*

It is essential that clinical education be viewed as part of the total educational experience in preparing personnel for allied health occupations. As Perry (1978, p. ix) pointed out: "Historically, allied health education has made the transition from total emphasis on hospital-based settings to emphasis on academic settings—sometimes without regard to the health care settings. We now realize that one cannot separate didactic instruction from clinical instruction as though they were two distinct entities. We must concentrate on partnership program development with integration of components as the key."

Integration of didactic and clinical education helps to bridge the gap between theory and practice and produces a multiplier effect—that is, by relating practice experiences to didactic materials, the effectiveness of both learning components is increased. Scanlan (1978) cites three levels at which the integration of didactic and clinical education must be achieved for maximum impact: administrative level, curriculum level, and course level.

The necessity for integration at the administrative level is clear. Continuity and articulation between clinical and didactic experiences depend on a clear understanding as to who is responsible for planning, content, and administration of clinical education. If students are left to their own devices in obtaining and pursuing clinical learning opportunities, there is no assurance that the quality and range of clinical experience is an adequate complement of the didactic experience.

Planning and assuring well-integrated and effective clinical education is complicated by the fact that many programs have large networks of affiliations. The approximately 4,000 basic occupational programs surveyed by ASAHP in 1975-76 reported 37,000 such affiliations, an average of about 9 per program. Eight percent had 35 or more affiliations. Moreover, many of the allied health programs of the commission's academic health center survey panel had affiliations scattered across the country.

Lack of continuity is most likely when students receive clinical education that is not administratively or contractually related to the didactic education, but it may occur even when formal arrangements are made, if divided responsibility results in failure to collaborate in developing an integrated total educational process. Although the specifics of how clinical and didactic education should be integrated and coordinated must be left to the institutions involved, there is a need for educational institutions to take on the responsibility of ensuring continuity and quality of the educational experience throughout the various phases of preparation.

7.1: *Educational institutions, which offer the didactic portion of an allied health program, should be responsible for the total education to ensure better integration of didactic and clinical education and sufficient breadth of clinical experiences; however, they must share the responsibility for planning, management, implementation, and evaluation with their clinical affiliates.*

7.2: *A written agreement should be formulated between the educational institution and each agency utilized for clinical education for the purpose of delineating objectives, authorities, responsibilities, and relationships.*

The best approaches to integration at the curriculum and course levels may vary by occupation. Theoretically, an approach that permits clinical experiences to be interspersed with didactic ones should be more effective than the old lock-step sequence in which all coursework is completed before students are exposed to the practice setting. Clinical experiences that are interspersed should help to illustrate, on a continuing basis, relationships between aspects of theory and practice. Moreover, early clinical exposure should help students reality-test their vocational choices and discover, before lengthy investment in coursework, any personal incompatibility with health care environments.

Unfortunately, very little research has been conducted to test these assumptions. Thus the commission does not feel justified in making recommendations on learning sequences. Instead, the need to study this topic is addressed in a subsequent recommendation dealing with research in clinical education. In the absence of proven effective guidelines, the commission believes that the best sequencing of didactic and clinical learning can be achieved in individual programs by ensuring that educators themselves have an understanding of the goals and processes of both components and of the need to integrate these components.

In many cases, different individuals are responsible for the academic and clinical phase of a student's preparation as a health professional. Full integration of a student's academic and clinical learning requires that the objectives of clinical education be well defined and understood and that these objectives reflect the goals of the educational institution as well as of practice needs. Faculty within the academic setting should be clinically current. The knowledge explosion, increasing specialization, and rapidly changing technology place great demands on academic faculty to update their clinical skills. Faculty within the clinical setting should be familiar with students' study programs and knowledge attainment so that maximum profit can be gained from the clinical experience.

7.3: *Educational institutions and clinical facilities should collaborate, or reevaluate current collaborative arrangements, to increase integration and improvement of clinical and didactic instruction through procedures such as:*

a. academic appointments for faculty responsible for planning and supervising clinical instruction
b. mechanisms to permit academic faculty to remain clinically current
c. organized joint planning for the overall curriculum by clinical and academic faculty
d. involvement of master clinicians in overall curriculum development
e. collaboration with health service providers to secure relevant preceptorships for and facilitate placement of graduate students

7.4: *Formal degree programs as well as continuing education programs should be designed specifically to prepare faculty to plan, supervise, and evaluate clinical practice.*

- Programs to prepare allied health faculty should include study of both clinical and didactic education and include courses in classroom teaching as well as practicum supervision.
- Educational institutions and professional organizations should develop continuing education courses and workshops on integrating clinical and didactic education for clinicians currently engaged in practicum supervision and academic faculty.

Although the settings for clinical practicum vary by occupational category, data from the 1975-76 ASAHP inventory of collegiate programs show that, overall, programs rely heavily on hospitals. Of those programs that report clinical affiliations, three out of four are affiliated with hospitals (Anderson and others, 1978, p. 23). Moreover, half of the programs have just one type of clinical affiliation. Clearly, many students are being offered only a limited exposure to the range of settings and delivery modes to which their competencies might be appropriately applied.

As described in Chapter Three, health services and settings are changing. Although the overall demand for allied health personnel in hospitals is not expected to decline in the near future, the areas of greatest growth in demand will be elsewhere. "New" settings, where certain categories of allied health personnel should find increasing opportunities, include organized group practices and ambulatory settings of various kinds, as well as clinics in business and industry. According to the ASAHP data, only 17 percent of programs provide experiences in outpatient clinics; moreover, the data do not show whether these clinics include settings, such as health maintenance organizations or holistic health centers, that would afford students a different perspective on health care from that which might be gained in the traditional hospital outpatient clinic. No information was obtained on any clinical practicum in industry.

Although increasing the range of clinical practicum sites has important implications for the quality of education, it also has some practical implications. Some institutions are experiencing difficulty in arranging clinical placements for their students because of requirements that clinical settings account for the costs of education separately from those of health services.

> 7.5: *Educational institutions should increase the use of the broad array of clinical patterns and sites to enhance both the clinical practicum and future job placement of clinical trainees.*

Moreover, expanding the clinical practicum methods and tools by further development of materials that can be used in a classroom setting would increase students' opportunities for translating theory into practice in all stages of a program. Such materials also would be useful for continuing education in remote areas where practitioners have limited access to advanced technology. Alternative learning methods should not completely substitute for education in actual practice settings but should be used to enhance and enlarge practical learning opportunities.

7.6: *Various methods of learning for clinical competence should be developed in sites other than patient health service facilities. These may include simulated clinical learning programs, programmed laboratory experiences, and other patient/client service areas.* Private foundations and the federal government should provide funds for development and demonstration of alternative methods of learning for clinical competence. Results of these demonstration projects should be widely disseminated.

Recommendation 8: *Research in clinical education methods and theory must be greatly expanded.*

The clinical practicum is generally believed to be an essential component of professional preparation. The commission has found, however, that little work has been done to determine what learning can be best accomplished in a practicum situation, how much clinical experience a student requires to attain minimum competence for safe and effective practice, which sites are needed for most relevant clinical experience, or what pattern of clinical education is most effective and/or cost-efficient.

8.1: *Intensive research on methods of clinical education should be conducted:*

a. to identify the types of professional learning that are most dependent on practical experiences
b. to validate or modify existing standards for the amount and type of clinical experience required for program accreditation and/or practitioner certification
c. to develop valid methods of measuring the cost of the clinical practicum
d. to evaluate the clinical education to determine that the objectives have been achieved
e. to determine the relative cost-effectiveness of different patterns of clinical education, including different sequencing of clinical and didactic components

This research should be conducted collaboratively by academic program faculty and clinical practicum supervisors, and whenever possible it should be done through interinstitutional arrangements or professional organization projects that promote sharing of efforts and findings. A center, such as one of the regional research centers whose establishment is recommended by this commission (see Corollary 10.3), should serve as a clearinghouse for sharing the results of these research efforts. Funds should be provided in future years for implementation of the most promising approaches.

Building the Capability for Leadership and Innovation

A recurring theme in this report is the important leadership role allied health practitioners, administrators, and educators can play in meeting the changing health service needs and priorities of this nation. Allied health personnel can contribute significantly to improve accessibility, continuity, and quality of health care, as well as to cost containment. Their services are particularly relevant to new national concerns and priorities. They have the flexibility and progressive spirit to lead the nation toward preventive care, health promotion, and integrated health services.

In order for the public to profit most from the potential contributions of the allied health occupations, greater emphasis must be placed on the development of leadership and research capabilities. Leadership development is critical in three areas: clinical leadership, planning and management leadership, and educational leadership. Research is needed for continued innovation and improvement in allied health services and in the educational processes that prepare those who will deliver the services. The commission is convinced that the human potential in the allied health occupations and disciplines is great and that it can be fully exploited for the ultimate goal of more cost-effective health services only if adequate funding for leadership, research, and innovative activities can be secured. Finally, in developing leadership in allied health education, attention should be given to the importance of role models for women and ethnic minorities.

The commission recommendations in this section are directed at achieving these major goals related to leadership development in allied health:

- strengthening preparation for clinical leadership
- strengthening preparation for planning and management of health services
- strengthening preparation for educational leadership
- increasing scholarly and research activities
- increasing representation of minorities and women in leadership

The commission believes that future improvements in allied health education and services require stronger commitment to leadership development by universities, health service providers, and professional associations.

> **Recommendation 9:** *The development of leadership in the clinical, managerial, and educational areas should be a priority for allied health education.*

The specialized body of knowledge associated with most allied health disciplines has been expanding rapidly. Curriculum design for *basic* occupational preparation can accommodate only a selected portion of all the theory and skills that might be useful to clinicians in the field. To incorporate all of the knowledge would result in an increased length of time for basic preparation and would have a negative effect on costs and availability of services. However, allied health clinicians desiring to have specialized knowledge in their field and to become master clinicians should have available the necessary formal mechanisms to achieve their goals.

Master clinicians provide direct care for patients whose problems are particularly complex, participate in clinical research, establish programs of service in nontraditional settings, and provide consultation, supervision, and on-the-job training for less experienced colleagues. In the past, most master clinicians have developed these skills largely through on-the-job experience and independent study. The commission believes that formal academic preparation helps to condense the time required to gain these skills and to enhance the mastery gained through practice.

Although many allied health disciplines have developed advanced-level academic degree and continuing education programs, these have often emphasized preparation for administration and teaching. The Bureau of Health Manpower has played a major role in supporting advanced education, but its grant program does not address the need for preparing clinical specialists, clinical investigators, or master clinicians because P.L. 94-484, Section 797(A), targets the advanced training support to teachers, administrators, and supervisors.

> 9.1: *Public agencies and private foundations should support qualified universities to develop advanced programs on a pilot or demonstration project basis for preparation of master clinicians.*
>
> - Programs for preparation of master clinicians should give more emphasis to the study of: (a) advanced clinical theory and method in the allied health discipline, and (b) methods of clinical research applicable to that discipline.
> - Programs for preparation of master clinicians should include an advanced level practicum. Public agencies and private foundations should support qualified specialized clinical service facilities to offer clinical preceptorships on a pilot or demonstration project basis to prepare master clinicians.
> - Any process of credentialing master clinicians should focus on the competencies essential for practice and recognize that they may be gained through academic preparation and/or on-the-job experience.

Allied health personnel collectively provide a large volume of services. The cost per unit of service is relatively low, but the total annual expenditure for these services contributes substantially to the national health bill. Because of the rising costs of health care services, continuous effort is needed to study the cost, quality, and effectiveness of allied health services. Relatively few of the procedures used by clinicians have been rigorously tested to determine their actual effectiveness in terms of quality of care and cost to the consumer. Such research is needed to establish valid guidelines for use of procedures by all clinicians.

9.2: *Qualified universities and health service organizations should conduct carefully controlled studies of the effect of clinicians on the cost and effectiveness of allied health services.*

- Master clinicians should provide leadership in planning and carrying out the needed clinical research.
- Both clinical and academic faculty should increase their efforts to test the clinical theories they teach.

Allied health faculty, on the one hand, may have the skills necessary to design worthwhile clinical research but often lack ready access to clinical facilities and patients. Many clinicians, on the other hand, lack expertise in research methods and access to needed library and other support facilities. An appropriate location for applied research could be in clinics and other agencies outside the university that have adopted a research mission. These clinics or agencies could serve as field stations for universities and clinical institutions, modeled after the land-grant university cooperative extension program in agriculture.

9.3: *"Field stations" should be established on a demonstration or trial basis to increase the volume, quality, relevance, and utilization of research in allied health clinical services.*

- University-based allied health units and clinical institutions should collaborate to develop trial "field stations" for clinical research providing necessary library, clinical, and other resources and a "critical mass" of scholars. In many cases, the studies should be interdisciplinary and interinstitutional.

- Financial support for these trial projects should be provided by federal agencies, private foundations, and other funding sources interested in allied health services and education.
- The effectiveness and feasibility of allied health clinical research "field stations" should be evaluated by university-based allied health schools and the results of such evaluations disseminated.

Effective application of established principles of health service planning and management could help to control the costs of health care and improve accessibility of allied health services. The commission believes a need exists for an increased effort to prepare persons in allied health occupations as effective health service planners and managers working in health service and community agencies, professional organizations, and academic institutions. Currently, only a few allied health personnel are actively involved in middle- and upper-level institutional or organizational decision making related to their services. The commission believes that it is essential for more allied health practitioners to have the requisite skills to assume a more active role in the planning and management of their services.

> 9.4: *Educational institutions, professional organizations, employers, and others should initiate, provide, and/or support programs of continuing education to teach planning and management skills to allied health personnel already in practice.* These should include: (a) circuit-riding courses for practitioners in rural areas, and (b) collaborative programs of staff education for small employers. Such instruction in planning and management skills should be interdisciplinary whenever possible.

A decade ago, the rapid expansion of allied health programs in collegiate institutions introduced a shortage of qualified faculty. Most of the health practitioners who were training allied health personnel in hospitals and other health care delivery settings lacked academic credentials and had little or no formal training in education. The needs of the proliferating programs were met by "faculty raiding, crash programs in instant pedagogy to convert health practitioners into instructors, hurried curriculum construction, and a widespread practice of recruiting inexperienced instructors" (W. K. Kellogg Foundation, 1977, p. 2).

During the last ten years, numerous programs were implemented to improve teaching and administrative skills. However, lack of relevant data on a national scale makes it difficult to assess what progress has been made. A number of program directors responding to a commission survey in 1977 stated that finding qualified faculty and administrators still constituted a major problem for allied health education. Faculty members were said to "teach as they were taught rather than striving to develop their role as educators" (Holmstrom, Bisconti, and Kent, 1978, p. 266). Cited as a major cause of the problem was the scarcity of graduate or teacher education programs in allied health. The need for continuing education programs for faculty members, for regional workshops to upgrade and update staff, and for the development of the capacity to do interdisciplinary research were all mentioned.

The commission supports the ongoing efforts to improve teaching and administrative skills. Other recommendations in this chapter include the suggestion that additional attention in faculty development programs be given to: (a) incorporation in the curriculum of subject matter relating to human values, prevention, and delivery systems; (b) use of role delineation studies in curriculum development; (c) use of methods to facilitate articulation and minimize unnecessary duplication of learning—such as modularized courses, specification and reporting of practice-based performance objectives, and flexible scheduling; and (d) sensitivity to the problems of disadvantaged minorities and methods of increasing their representation in allied health education.

The need for allied health education to participate more fully in the life of the total educational institution has not been systematically addressed. This need is particularly critical in colleges and universities, where the majority of allied health programs are housed. Without such involvement, allied health education components remain outside the mainstream of campus life, and this isolation may be reflected in a continued lack of understanding and recognition of the allied health occupations and the importance of the services they provide. Isolation may result from organizational patterns and structures, physical location of programs, or intrainstitutional differentiation in faculty titles, qualifications, orientation, rank, benefits, and salary; it may also result from insufficient knowledge on the part of faculty and administrators of these programs of the history, structure, issues, and trends of American higher education.

9.5: *Programs to prepare allied health faculty should include:*

a. the study of history and philosophy of higher education
b. a knowledge of health care delivery
c. research methodology and ways it can be applied in day-to-day teaching
d. interdisciplinary processes
e. instructional methods, especially as they apply to clinical settings and direct patient care
f. advanced study and methods in each clinical field
g. coursework in curriculum development and planning

Recommendation 10: *Support for research on allied health education should be substantially increased, and allied health faculty should be encouraged to strengthen their commitment to research.*

In order to develop the quality and strength of allied health units in collegiate institutions and build the knowledge base for allied health education and practice, substantial scholarly activity must be undertaken by some of the faculty. Likewise, in order to develop scholarly activity there must be an appropriate reward system.

10.1: *Administrators of allied health programs should regard scholarly activity as a necessary part of the* *total activities of faculty and take this into account in determining faculty needs, budgeting, and selection and promotion of faculty.*

10.2: *Faculty development institutes and workshops should include sessions on research and writing.*

The need for research relating to allied health education and services is critical. This commission was hampered at every turn by the lack of data to answer policy questions and to test assumptions. Particularly needed are studies on the following topics:

- *Cost-effectiveness of educational processes.* There is no information available today on what constitutes a cost-effective program in allied health. Even cost accounting methodology is in the pioneering stage (see Corollary 14.4). Moreover, the criteria for measuring effectiveness still need to be determined and operationalized.
- *Impact of institutional environments and program characteristics on students.* No systematic longitudinal studies of students in allied health occupations are being conducted nationally. Without student data, it is impossible to determine what the impact of the various settings and educational processes on student progress may be. Even the basic assumption on which the allied health education concepts rest—the value of clustering health occupations programs rather than preparing students in isolated units—remains untested.

  Student selection and counseling processes in allied health are conducted today in an information vacuum. Because of the high student demand for majors that will provide marketable skills, it is often possible for allied health programs to select students with top grades. Heavy reliance on grades as the primary selection criterion may result in the exclusion of persons from disadvantaged backgrounds, including minority students who might eventually help to fill the health service gaps in urban underserved areas. It may result also in the exclusion of persons who are best suited for the occupation. Students choosing different health occupations also differ in terms of their demographic backgrounds as well as their attitudes and value systems (Holmstrom, Knepper, and Kent, 1977, a, b, c). Top grades do not necessarily predict adjustment to the demands of particular health careers. For some disciplines, other personal characteristics may be much more important predictors of achievement and satisfaction in the program and on the job.

For studies of institutional and program impact, ongoing surveys such as the ASAHP Collegiate Inventory can serve as a useful base, but they should be expanded to include more questions on the institutional environment and educational processes. Student data, of course, are essential.

- *Faculty characteristics.* Very little information is available today on allied health faculty, their backgrounds, goals, scholarly productivity, and continuing development needs. Such information is necessary to ensure that faculty development programs are appropriately targeted. In addition, the traditional criteria for hiring and promoting faculty in higher education, such as degrees and scholarly productivity, may not be associated with teacher effectiveness in all allied health subject areas. Because allied health education has such a significant and direct impact on the well-being of the public, it is important to identify faculty characteristics that promote student development in various knowledge and skill areas.
- *Relating education to service needs.* Numerous questions concerning the relation of education to service needs should be addressed through major research studies. Chief among these questions is how best to meet the pressing health manpower needs of rural and urban underserved areas.

These major national research efforts require a research capability of a magnitude that is yet to be developed in allied health education settings. The development of research centers with the requisite capabilities should be planned in a way that will provide the greatest service to the broad interests in allied health education. Centers distributed in broad interstate regions could serve as clearinghouses for information which, as discussed previously, is critically needed for planning educational programs that meet health service needs. They could also serve as settings for preparing future allied health leaders in research methodology and could provide guidance and technical assistance.

> **10.3:** *Public and private funds should support five or six regional centers for research and development in allied health.* Such centers should be based in a university with a school of allied health or in another qualified organization with a strong institutional commitment to allied health. They should: (a) serve as resource centers for individual institutions seeking research guidance; (b) make state and regional manpower data available, either by analyzing nationally collected data or by collecting new data; (c) develop broad information storage and research capabilities, with each center specializing in different problem areas; (d) conduct national research studies on allied health education topics; and (e) provide opportunities for preceptorships in research. Centers should coordinate activities through an Executive Council to ensure comparability of methodologies used in data collection and reporting and to avoid unnecessary duplication of effort, particularly with respect to area of specialization.

> **Recommendation 11:** *Educational institutions should strengthen their efforts to increase the representation of minorities and women in leadership positions.*

As described in Chapter Four, women constitute the majority among students and practitioners in many allied health occupations but a minority among leaders. One reason is that many of today's leaders (both clinical and in education) were prepared in disciplines other than allied health. Another reason is that a relatively small proportion of recent doctoral recipients in allied health occupations were women. Ethnic minorities are also underrepresented, relative to their proportion of the total U.S. population, in allied health education in general and in leadership positions in particular. As a result, there are very few role models for minorities and women among the current cadre of leaders in allied health education and services. Although there are no national data on allied health faculty, tentatively, one in ten of those employed in colleges and universities may belong to an ethnic minority group. In the NCAHE survey of eighty academic and seventy-three clinical leaders, only two clinical leaders and eight academic leaders were minority-group members: three blacks, two Asian-Americans, two Hispanic-Americans, and one American Indian. Further, very few of the leaders were women. Research findings on equal opportunity and discrimination have shown that solid credentials and participation in the "buddy system" are very effective ways of entering power positions for those who have previously been excluded from such positions. Leadership development programs, particularly such prestigious ones as those given by the American Council on Education, provide an opportunity for women and minorities to become participants in the "buddy system" which includes the leaders of the future.

> 11.1: *Women and minorities should be encouraged to pursue advanced degrees and participate in leadership development programs.*

Planning and Administration: Diversity Without Waste

This commission does not encourage a monolithic approach to allied health education. On the contrary, the commission believes that variety promotes the innovativeness and growth that is essential for progress—perhaps even for survival. At the same time, we can no longer afford the luxury of waste. Thus the planning and administration of allied health programs should be based on principles that encourage variety or diversity but discourage inefficiency. The recommendations in this section are addressed to three kinds of excess associated with aspects of planning and administration. The first results when programs that do not meet health service demands or are not needed are either established or continued. The second results when educational processes are unnecessarily duplicated and resources are used inefficiently. The third results when planning and administration for each separate program take place in a vacuum, without benefit of shared methodologies, experiences, and knowledge. In addition, faulty student selection procedures and inadequate counseling may result in student attrition, wasting both educational and human resources.

The commission recommendations in this section are directed at achieving these major goals related to maintaining the current diversity in educational settings and programs in allied health but without waste:

- developing objective criteria for program establishment, expansion, and termination
- improving articulation
- improving student opportunities, particularly for minorities
- strengthening information sharing and interaction

> **Recommendation 12:** *The establishment, expansion, maintenance, reduction, and termination of allied health programs should be based on manpower requirements, adequacy and efficient use of available resources, and collaboration within and among educational and other institutions.*

Some types of educational settings, such as private career schools, hospitals, and the military, are particularly attuned to manpower needs. They have the flexibility to initiate and terminate programs with relatively little time lag in response to their own requirements for health personnel or those of local employers. Such flexibility is not typical of collegiate settings, however. Once programs are established, they are not easily phased out; thus the need for analysis is especially critical in the collegiate sector, both prior to program establishment and throughout the life of the program.

Although the planning of collegiate allied health programs is becoming increasingly subject to state and regional controls (as reported in Chapter Five), the commission believes that close public scrutiny does not lessen the importance of self-regulation. Responsible decision making on the part of all concerned in planning and administration of allied health programs is necessary so that programs are established and maintained (1) as a reflection of manpower requirements, (2) with assurance of adequate institutional resources, and (3) with the best use of existing resources through collaboration and sharing.

There has been much concern expressed over duplication in allied health education. Duplication in itself is not wasteful and may be necessary to preserve diversity. Thus the commission does not find the presence in a given geographic area of more than one program for the same occupation unwarranted, as long as each program is meeting health service needs. However, unnecessary duplication of educational resources and processes resulting from the isolation and lack of coordination of components is wasteful.

The commission believes that allied health program directors should develop arrangements both within and between institutions for sharing specialized institutional resources. Such resources may include physical resources, human resources (faculty and students), and clinical facilities. Such arrangements should be considered in all stages of program planning and administration, not just at the time of program establishment, as a way of increasing the efficiency and effectiveness of the program.

As described in Chapter Five, collaborative arrangements between institutions have been guided by several purposes: (1) to meet special manpower needs such as those of rural areas; (2) to meet program needs for expensive equipment and facilities without unnecessary duplication of resources, and (3) to provide opportunities for the transition from one program to another without unnecessary duplication of learning. One of the most promising collaborative models for meeting the needs of medically underserved areas is the urban-rural linkage model, which links remote educational institutions with an urban institution that has substantial existing resources for instruction in health fields. Other promising approaches described in Chapter Five for meeting special manpower needs include collaboration to meet short-term needs, intensive training in national or regional centers, and student exchange contracts.

Entering into collaboration as a means of shoring up weak programs is often not a good policy. Collaborative arrangements are likely to be more successful when participants enter the arrangement from positions of strength. Particularly for allied health education, problems such as low enrollments and difficulty in placing graduates should be viewed as possible indicators that the program is no longer needed. In such cases, collaborative arrangements should be considered only if they would enable the redirection of institutional resources to different geographical areas where the demand for graduates is greater.

12.1: *In establishing new programs and evaluating existing ones, consideration should be given to the different service areas of different types of institutions: State-controlled institutions in general must attempt to relate their production of health personnel to state or regional requirements. Private institutions—both nonprofit and proprietary—must develop programs that meet the requirements of their service area; for private nonprofit institutions the service area may not be geographically defined, whereas for proprietary institutions the service area will probably be local.*

12.2: *Market analysis techniques should be used to advise program directors and school administrators of the employer demand primarily and the attractiveness to students secondarily.*

12.3: *Alternatives to establishing new programs to meet manpower requirements should be developed, especially when the additional supply requirements are small or likely to be saturated after a short time period. Such alternatives may include:*

- alternative service delivery modes to improve distribution of personnel (for example, to bring services of existing personnel to underserved rural areas)

- expansion of existing programs
- extension of existing capabilities to other geographical areas (such as the urban-rural extension model)
- short intensive programs in regional centers that have appropriate capabilities
- student and/or faculty exchange
- cooperative arrangements for rotating programs, which move periodically as the need is saturated, or for programs with built-in termination dates

12.4: *As a criterion for establishing and continuing programs, educational institutions must assure:*

- the adequacy of clinical affiliations and that students receive appropriate clinical practicum (see Recommendation 7 and Corollaries 7.1 to 7.6).
- sufficient funds to continue a new program through at least two completing classes.

12.5: *Efforts should be made to utilize existing community resources and collaborate with other institutions (both educational and clinical) that already have programs in place or that have some of the required resources.*

12.6: *Arrangements should be made for maximum use of existing institutional resources, including shared courses.* In particular, whenever possible, allied health students should receive instruction in the basic sciences and humanities through participation in general university courses offered by faculty of the department in those disciplines rather than in special courses offered exclusively for allied health majors.

12.7: *If fewer than four out of five graduates who seek employment in the occupation for which they prepared succeed in finding employment, the program should be terminated unless there is reasonable assurance of continuing need for a reduced number of graduates and the number of students enrolled can be reduced without affecting the quality of education.*

12.8: *New doctoral programs for health occupations should be developed only if existing doctoral programs in basic sciences or other fields do not meet the needs for production of persons with doctoral-level competencies.*

12.9: *Funds should be provided by the federal government or private foundations to a statewide coordinating agency such as the Southern Regional Education Board for a two-stage project to increase the use by educational institutions and state and regional agencies of guidelines based on the considerations previously outlined.*

Stage One—Conference on allied health education program establishment and continuing review. Participants in this conference should include educators, state planners, selected members of the higher education board of each state, representatives from HSAs and from regional and national higher education associations. Discussion leaders should include persons with expertise on topics to be considered (for example, manpower studies, market analyses, alternatives to program establishment). By working in small groups, conference participants should develop guidelines for program establishment and review based upon the considerations recommended by this commission.

Stage Two—Paid Consultancies. A list of allied health programs that have successfully implemented approaches relevant to considerations listed in Corollaries 12.3, 12.5, and 12.6 should be compiled and funds provided to pay for consultants from these programs to help implement these approaches in other institutions.

Recommendation 13: *Educational and collaborating institutions should adopt mechanisms to facilitate the removal of unnecessary barriers to student progress.*

The word *articulation* with reference to education is commonly used to describe "the series of activities accompanying the move from one institution to another" (Kintzer, 1976, p. 1). One aspect of articulation, problems associated with transfer of credit from two-year to four-year colleges, has been studied extensively. Here the word *articulation* is used in the broader and more active sense conveyed by the definition in Webster's *New Collegiate Dictionary,* "the action or manner of jointing or interrelating," and refers to all components of learning.

Continuity between various educational levels and study disciplines benefits society and the consumer of education. It is cost-effective to include in each phase of education only those aspects of required learning that have not already been attained; it is wasteful for society to pay for unnecessary repetition of learning experiences. It is wasteful also to attempt to teach advanced knowledge and skills to students who have not already attained the basic competencies on which the advanced knowledge and skills should be built.

For effective health service, personnel at various levels are needed; society cannot afford a health system composed solely of "chiefs." Moreover, not all students have the aptitude or interest to move up a career ladder and not everyone should be encouraged to do so. Nevertheless, in a rapidly changing health industry, mechanisms to facilitate career changes are necessary for optimal flexibility of the health workforce. Redirecting the talents of existing practitioners from obsolete or low-demand services to new or high-demand services is cost-effective. It requires lower educational expenditures than preparing new students, improves the utilization of health practitioners, and avoids unnecessary expansion of the health workforce.

Providing maximum opportunity for student development without added cost to society can be achieved by removing arbitrary barriers in the accreditation and credentialing processes and the educational system that impede smooth articulation and transfer of credit, and by providing recognition for learning that has already taken place. In collegiate settings, such recognition takes the form of credit or waiver of requirements.

The North Carolina study of articulation and transfer of credit in allied health education identified three basic articulation models involving collegiate institutions (Boatman and Huther, 1974):

- Model A: from preprofessional to professional curricula (the standard model for medical technologists, physical therapists, and other occupations).
- Model B: from an associate degree basic occupational preparation program to a baccalaureate program preparing students for expanded functions in the same occupation (sometimes referred to as the "inverted" curriculum since general education preparation follows professional preparation, often involving programs in dental hygiene, respiratory therapy, and radiologic technology).
- Model C: from an associate degree basic occupational preparation program to a baccalaureate basic occupational program for a higher-level occupational title in the same discipline (for example, from medical laboratory technician to medical technologist, medical record technician to medical record administrator, dietetic technician to dietitian). Referred to as the two-plus-two model.

Although these three models are the most common and have received the most attention, they are not the only ones. Other articulation patterns include:

- from certificate to associate programs
- from bachelor's to graduate programs (a) in the same discipline and (b) in education, administration, or basic sciences
- from an occupational preparation program in one discipline to an occupational preparation program in another discipline
- from an occupational preparation program to general studies (for enrichment)
- interinstitutional transfer within the same major
- nontraditional transfer (applicants who bring knowledge and skills acquired in a noncollegiate setting; applicants with old records)

In spite of a national trend toward more flexible admissions and transfer policies, many allied health programs continue to be rigid and do not permit exemption of students from specific portions of the curriculum, even though they have demonstrated competency in their areas. Such inflexibility results in inefficiency and represents an insurmountable burden to employed persons who wish to pursue further education. Even the community college, which historically has served the needs of adult learners, does not appear to be providing significant opportunities for part-time study for allied health occupations. In 1976, 86 percent of students in two-year college allied health programs were enrolled on a full-time basis—an identical proportion to that within four-year colleges and universities.

Institutional commitment to flexible scheduling and exemption of students from portions of a program is inhibited by state formula funding policies that encourage full-time enrollments (this problem is addressed in Corollary 15.2). However, many institutional barriers result simply because administrators do not have the tools to make articulation work. Few programs have developed learning modules based on components of practice. Few have developed instruments to assess what students have already learned and what they still need to learn. Without such knowledge, it is difficult to plan a program that builds new learning on old learning effectively. Performance objectives for courses often have not been clearly stated and reported. Thus it is difficult to relate what has been learned in the past to what the program seeks to teach. Transcripts reporting letter grades give little indication of the performance objectives attained by students in courses.

13.1: *Efforts to improve articulation should include the following:*

a. use of equivalency examinations and other assessment tools for identifying objectives already attained and still to be attained
b. modularization of courses with waiver of portions that duplicate prior learning experiences

c. specification of practice-based performance objectives and reporting attainment of specified objectives
d. flexible scheduling and other approaches enabling persons already working in allied health occupations to study on a part-time basis

Some institutions and state systems already have taken steps to remove these barriers and have developed innovative approaches to minimize unnecessary duplication of learning. The lessons learned from these approaches should be shared as the basis for broader implementation of administrative policies and procedures that facilitate articulation.

13.2: *Allied health administrators should take the responsibility for comparing their own programs' content and structure with that of other programs that have been successful in facilitating articulation. Faculty development programs should include instruction in these methods.*

13.3: *ASAHP should sponsor a national conference on articulation with problem-solving workshops.* In planning the conference, the experiences and results of other conferences on articulation (for example, the Airlie House Conference on Articulation in postsecondary education in general and the State of Virginia conference on articulation in allied health education) should be studied. Conference participants should include representatives of professional associations, higher education boards, HSAs, and all types of educational institutions described in the commission report. Discussion leaders should include representatives of programs that have successfully implemented approaches to facilitate articulation.

The proceedings and conclusions, including model approaches deemed promising by conference participants, should be broadly disseminated. Funds should then be awarded for consultants from programs that have implemented promising approaches to assist other institutions initiating similar projects.

13.4: *Funds should be provided to develop nationally recognized equivalency exams, similar to those of the College Level Examination Program, for allied health education subject matter of a multidisciplinary nature (for example, anatomy, medical terminology).*

Since allied health education has as its goals the preparation of competent practitioners, articulation between educational levels or disciplines is influenced by articulation between practice levels and occupations. Because of the complexities of occupational patterns in the health fields, career options need to be delineated for each occupation, and attention needs to be given to the specific articulation problem of each.

13.5: *Professional associations should take the lead in delineating career options for the occupations they represent and identifying ways of facilitating career advancement and change.* They should conduct follow-up studies of graduates to monitor their educational and career progress and to identify barriers, and they should use the role delineation study groups to find ways of improving interoccupational articulation. (See Corollary 2.1.)

Possible barriers to articulation inherent in accreditation processes have recently come under scrutiny at the national level. According to the Joint Statement on Transfer and Award of Academic Credit approved by the Council on Postsecondary Accreditation, the American Council on Education, and the American Association of Collegiate Registrars and Admissions Officers: "Transfer of credit from one institution to another involves at least three considerations: (1) the educational quality of the institution from which the student transfers; (2) the comparability of the nature, content, and level of credit earned to that offered by the receiving institution; and (3) the appropriateness and applicability of the credit earned to the programs offered by the receiving institution, in light of the student's educational goals" (Council on Postsecondary Accreditation, 1978, p. 1). The statement also notes that, currently, accreditation neglects the second and third considerations. The three associations indicate in this statement that "transfer-of-credit policies should encompass educational accomplishment attained in extrainstitutional settings" (p. 1). The commission encourages continued study of potential barriers, as well as self-scrutiny on the part of individual accrediting bodies. This self-scrutiny should go beyond the transfer-of-credit issues and address possible barriers to articulation in the various requirements for award of accreditation status.

13.6: *Accrediting bodies should examine their policies to determine if and how they may be obstructing articulation between levels and between disciplines.*

Graduates of allied health programs should have the opportunity to transfer to nonhealth programs to pursue education that is beyond what is required for practice but meets personal needs. Moreover, additional skills and knowledge for career advancement can be acquired by study in nonhealth disciplines. Cost savings to society can be achieved by utilizing existing educational programs in liberal arts, business, education, and other fields, where appropriate, rather than starting new programs that are customized for health practitioners. Today students who wish to transfer from an occupational program to an arts and sciences major or to another occupational major are likely to receive very little academic credit for the coursework they have already completed.

In order to provide an opportunity for qualified and motivated students to develop beyond the limits of the basic occupational program or to complete the prerequisites to pursue graduate study in related disciplines, some educational institutions are experimenting with a Bachelor of Health Science program of an interdisciplinary nature. These interdisciplinary programs prepare persons who have already completed basic occupational programs to perform advanced functions, and they do so without adding to the proliferation of advanced-level programs in separate disciplines. The model can be used to provide personal enrichment opportunities to students as well. In the University of Alabama program, plans of study will be developed with each student, based on the student's objectives. For example, if the student plans to enroll for graduate study, the study plan will include the necessary prerequisites.

> 13.7: *The three regional higher education boards should examine the feasibility of establishing regional Bachelor of Health Science programs to allow persons prepared in occupations that are not articulated with the bachelor's level the opportunity to pursue further study in humanities, social sciences, and/or natural sciences, as well as provide greater exposure on an interdisciplinary basis to health problems.* Current experimental programs should be examined. Funds should be provided for paid consultancies to help implement successful models in other institutions.

One aspect of the articulation process that starts before entry into postsecondary allied health education programs is the linking of vocational interests and aptitudes, early education, and choice of occupational program. Enrollment in an allied health program, unlike enrollment for liberal arts study, means a real commitment on the part of both the student and the program. A wrong choice resulting in dropping out hurts the student as well as the program. Similarly, a wrong choice resulting in failure to use the education in a health career is wasteful to all concerned. To ensure a better match between student's aptitudes and requirements of the program and the occupation, whenever possible students should receive accurate information on or exposure to allied health occupations during their high school years.

> 13.8: *Allied health administrators should establish links with local secondary school systems to inform stu-*

dents about allied health careers and requirements of educational programs and to encourage participation in work experiences in health settings during the high school years.

The concern among students today for acquiring marketable skills has greatly increased the attractiveness of occupationally oriented programs of study. Consequently, many programs have a large pool of applicants from which to choose. In 1975-76, the ratio of applicants to first-year enrollments was 2.1 to 1 in two-year college programs and 2.6 to 1 in four-year college programs. Moreover, the number of applicants per program increased between 1973-74 and 1975-76 by 5 percent in four-year colleges and universities and by 12 percent in two-year colleges (Anderson and others, 1978). Lacking selection criteria, program administrators may rely heavily on grades as an indicator of ability to complete coursework successfully. National data on college students show that those who majored in health disciplines were likely to have relatively high grades compared with students in other majors (Holmstrom, 1973). The growing importance of grades for admission to allied health programs discourages students from disadvantaged backgrounds whose high school achievement may not accurately reflect their intrinsic ability to become good health practitioners. Admissions criteria should be examined and reevaluated. Grades may correlate with completion of a course but may not predict success in practice. Studies should be carried out to determine the degree to which other criteria such as motivation, prior experience in health care, and personal traits such as independence and creativity should be considered in the selection of students. Such studies could be carried out by one of the regional research centers whose establishment is recommended (see Corollary 10.3).

In addition, in order to meet the health needs of diverse cultures and ethnic groups, an effort should be made to select students from different backgrounds. The commission found that the representation of black students in the allied health student population in 1975-76 (about 10 percent) was lower than the representation of blacks in the U.S. population (12 percent) and in the U.S. population aged eighteen to twenty-four (13 percent) (Bureau of the Census, 1975). Even more discouraging, they were substantially underrepresented in the pipeline for the relatively high-level allied health occupations and slightly overrepresented in the pipeline for those occupations requiring less training. Hispanic Americans also were more likely than white students to be working toward an associate degree or diploma and less likely to be working toward a baccalaureate or advanced degree.

> **13.9:** *Educational institutions, with the advice and counsel of professional associations and practitioners, should evaluate student selection procedures to determine whether more reliable indicators of probable academic success than those presently in use can be found and utilized.*

A good example of efforts to recruit blacks into allied health professions is the "Project Black Awareness-Health Careers" of the School of Community and Allied Health, University of Alabama in Birmingham. This project uses a multifaceted approach to inform, counsel, and recruit blacks into allied health programs. The project has been more successful in increasing the black to white ratio in associate degree/certificate level programs than in baccalaureate and graduate level programs (Pruitt and Ray, 1979). Part of the reason may be that the project had no funds for financial assistance. Recruitment efforts without financial and other support services are bound to have limited success. Most important, perhaps, are the attitudes of the faculty: An increased sensitivity to the problems of disadvantaged minorities is essential to retain and train these students for occupations that could put them in the mainstream of American life.

> **13.10:** *Recruitment efforts to increase minority representation in allied health programs should be strengthened through provision of counseling and finan-*

cial assistance. Training institutes for allied health faculty and administrators should include seminars dealing with the matter of minority student recruitment.

Special consideration should be given to the needs of some institutions that serve an important function in providing health manpower but have difficulty meeting the criteria for establishing and maintaining programs. The underrepresentation of minorities in allied health occupations contributes to the problem of some medically underserved populations. Traditionally black institutions are a major source of manpower, but administrators of allied health programs from some of these institutions have reported to the commission that securing clinical affiliation sites for their students is a serious problem. Other educational institutions and health care providers should collaborate to help traditionally black institutions overcome such difficulty (for example, following the model of the Eastern Virginia Health Education Consortium).

13.11: *It is imperative that hospitals, independent clinical laboratories, and other health service facilities provide clinical experiences to students of traditionally black institutions.*

Recommendation 14: *Information relating to administration and planning in allied health education should be collected and shared systematically.*

In the grass-roots survey conducted by commission staff as a means of tapping concerns and identifying topics to study, administrators expressed frustration at having to plan and administer programs in a vacuum. During the two-year study, commission staff received numerous phone calls from administrators with similar complaints who hoped to receive guidance regarding where to turn for data on various topics, model approaches, and persons with expertise in particular areas. Clearly, planning without benefit of the experiences of others leads to wasteful duplication of effort. The research centers recommended earlier should help to fill this critical information and guidance need. In addition, a national clearinghouse on allied health education literature should be established.

> 14.1: *ASAHP should seek funds from the National Institute of Education to establish an ERIC Clearinghouse on Allied Health Education.*

Current national data collection projects are of great value in making policy decisions of various kinds. Such projects include the ASAHP Inventory of Health Occupations Programs in Collegiate Settings, the AHA Survey of Health Occupations Training Programs in Hospitals, The U.S. Office of Education's Survey of Postsecondary Schools with Occupational Programs, and the surveys of the Cooperative Health Information System. Such surveys should be continued and expanded.

> 14.2: *A major thrust of the federal government's involvement in allied health education should be the systematic and continuous collection and dissemination of data on the numbers and distribution of health manpower in all occupational areas, including information on projected openings.* Such data should be reported regionally within states and made generally available.

> 14.3: *The federal government should continue to support biennial national inventories of allied health education programs.* These inventories should be extended to all educational settings described in the commission report and should be reported regionally within states and made generally available. In addition, future surveys should include questions on nontraditional approaches to education (for example, use of equivalency examinations, flexible scheduling, contract learning, external degrees), and ASAHP should publish a directory of programs using these approaches.

In order to maximize program cost-effectiveness, a uniform system of cost accounting should be developed and shared. This would provide administrators with normative data against which to measure their own programs and would help them identify practices that are not cost-effective; it would also be of value when considering future developments. In addition, a uniform system would provide valuable information to legislators, boards of governors, and others responsible for funding allied health programs.

> 14.4: *The federal government should provide funds to the National Center for Higher Education Management Systems (NCHEMS) and/or similar organizations for development of a system of cost accounting for allied health programs to identify actual program costs which could be translated into costs per student for use of educational institutions and for a study of comparative costs to be used by educational institutions and professional associations at local, state, and national levels.*

Another type of information sharing that has occurred only in the most limited way is international exchange. The range of allied health services in most countries varies from "paramedical aides" or "nurse auxiliaries" to "elementary doctor substitutes" and "primary health practitioners." Currently, the functional role of allied health workers in these countries is undergoing rapid change—somewhat comparable to what has happened in the United States—generally characterized by longer and more formal training. The utilization and types of allied health workers seem to depend on the supply of physicians, class distinctions, and, to a large extent, the philosophy of a nation's health service system with respect to the rights of the population to obtain medical care. The education of allied health workers reflects these differences as well as the overall educational system of each country and its resources (Roemer, 1976, pp. 203-209). Nonetheless, there are lessons to be learned from the experience of other countries. Similarly, allied health faculty, administrators, and practitioners in the United States have much to offer to program planners and administrators in other countries.

14.5: *Schools of allied health should be encouraged to arrange exchange programs with faculty from other countries.*

Finally, the most effective kind of information sharing often takes place in informal networks. Allied health administrators should seek to establish such networks and to take an active role in the broader planning processes. Particularly at the state and regional level, such involvement is critical so that persons with regulatory and funding authorities can acquire a better understanding of allied health education and benefit from experiences and knowledge of the educators.

14.6: *Administrators in allied health education programs for all levels of preparation should work closely with health planning and regulatory agencies, legislative bodies, and governing boards of academic institutions.*

Funding: Key to Future Progress

Recommendation 15: *Significantly increased funding for allied health should be provided at the federal, state, and local government levels and from private resources.*

If allied health services are essential to the well-being of the nation—and this commission believes they are—allied health education is equally essential. Allied health services depend on allied health education. The informally and haphazardly prepared health practitioner might have suited the level of sophistication of health care delivery at the turn of the century, but today the knowledge and skills required to perform health services are much more advanced. Formal education programs for most allied health occupations are the only means of ensuring that a sufficient number of personnel will be adequately prepared. Although some individuals may be able to acquire the necessary knowledge and skills by other means, most will require formal postsecondary preparation ranging from short-term training to graduate study. Moreover, the continued improvement of allied health services—in terms of quality, cost-effectiveness, access, and continuity—depends on allied health education. Without advanced programs and formal leadership development, it is unlikely that the necessary research and development activities would be conducted. Such research and development can be beneficial not only directly, by leading to improvement in services, but also indirectly, by improving educational processes so that practitioners are better prepared. The future of allied health services depends on financial support for allied health education.

The commission believes that funding for allied health has been minuscule in the past in comparison with contributions made to the health of the nation by allied health personnel. The commission recommends that all parties work together toward securing adequate and continuous funding for allied health education and services. Responsibilities of federal, state, and local governments, educational institutions, professional associations, and other interested groups differ, but they all share the major goal of keeping allied health a vital segment of the nation's health workforce.

Stability and continuity of financial support for programs in allied health must be assured by the educational institutions in order to maintain quality and increase the cost-effectiveness of educational processes. One of the major problems of many allied health programs has been their need to depend on project funds from relatively short-term federal grants or from foundation support. In many instances, programs of real significance have died when the foundation or government funds were no longer available. Some activities, such as faculty and leadership development, are too important to allow to go untended. These activities, which must be considered as continuing, cannot be adequately carried out unless institutional funds are available without diminishing support for regular teaching, research, and service functions. To make the best use of grant funds from foundations or other sources, institutional commitments following the start-up period are essential.

> 15.1: *Private and governmental funding agencies should require institutional commitment of funds, by the time the grant period ends, for projects that meet agreed-upon objectives.*

Many state coordinating or governing boards allocate funds to state institutions on the basis of numbers of full-time equivalent students, and it becomes almost impossible to fund special activities from state-appropriated funds. It is the position of the commission that state coordinating or governing boards should be "enablers" rather than "regulators." Greater flexibility could be built into state formulas for distributing funds to higher education institutions, thus permitting them to use state-appropriated funds for activities such as those that have been supported in the past through federal or foundation funds. Moreover, as discussed earlier, state formula funding policies based on full-time equivalent enrollments have a negative impact on cost containment because they create incentives for lengthening contact hours, and on articulation because they discourage flexible scheduling and such innovative approaches as the use of challenge exams to exempt students from repeating study of subject matter already mastered.

> 15.2: *States with formula funding policies based on full-time enrollments should reexamine their policies and seek ways to permit greater flexibility.* These policies should permit use of funds for special activities to improve the quality and cost-effectiveness of education. They should encourage flexible scheduling and part-time enrollment.

Allied health personnel provide a vast range of essential services. Because of the dynamic nature of health service delivery, the nation cannot afford a static educational system. Adequate funding is essential for the growth and development required to continue to prepare practitioners and leaders with the capabilities to meet health service needs effectively.

The significant contribution of allied health has not yet received appropriate recognition in funding policies relating to health manpower preparation. During the fiscal years 1957 through 1976, a total of $4.2 billion was appropriated by the federal government for health manpower education; only $183 million, just over 4 percent, was allocated to allied health education. The extent of this imbalance in funding imperatives is even more dramatic in light of the fact that individuals involved in allied health occupations compose a significant portion of the nation's total health manpower, and that the appropriate use of allied health practitioners can produce substantial health care cost economies and extend the reach of available health care services to the traditionally unserved and underserved areas of this country.

It has been stated that allied health education is a resource for the community, state, and nation. The responsibility of the federal government is to provide the necessary support to assure that priorities are met at the national level.

15.3. *The federal government should continue to provide funds for national data collection on allied health education and manpower.* Inventories of educational programs should be expanded to include noncollegiate and nonhospital programs.

15.4: *The federal government should provide adequate funds to support research activities in allied health education and services.* Such activities should include:

a. Establishment of a longitudinal data base on students to assess the impact of institutional and program characteristics on student progress and to monitor trends in the characteristics and goals of the student pool.
b. Systematic collection of information on allied health faculty to determine faculty development needs.
c. Assessment of contributions of allied health personnel to meeting various national health priorities (for example, bringing services to underserved areas, cost containment).
d. Application of role delineation studies to education, including establishment of commonalities in service functions and educational needs.
e. Studies to improve the quality and cost-effectiveness of allied health education and services.
f. Clinical research in allied health services.

15.5: *The federal government should also provide adequate funds for student aid programs and special projects for the disadvantaged and disabled to accomplish the national goals of equal access to allied health education and improving health care for medically unserved or underserved groups.*

Finally, the implementation of many of the recommendations in this report is linked to federal support. Private foundations have contributed significantly to the development of allied health education and services and, it is hoped, will continue their invaluable support in the future. However, it would be unfortunate if the federal government did not assume its share of the responsibility and relied on the states or private foundations to carry the burden alone. Further, the funding of allied health education by the federal government has been extremely inadequate in the past and needs to be strengthened.

15.7: *Federal funding of allied health education should be increased and maintained at a level consistent with contributions made to the health of the nation by allied health personnel.*

There is consensus that funds for special projects to improve the quality and cost-effectiveness of allied health education in future years will be scarce. No longer can those involved in allied health education count on easily won support. Raising adequate funds to move forward in the next decade will require a real commitment to active fund raising on the part of allied health educators, administrators, and professional groups individually and in organized alliances, all of whom will be forced to look beyond traditional funding sources. Although techniques, such as proposal writing, may need strengthening, much broader problems in fund seeking need to be addressed.

15.8: *ASAHP and its state chapters should arrange for experts in fund raising for allied health education projects to conduct workshops on the topic in conjunction with national and local allied health meetings.* The names of individuals who can provide reliable information based on sound experience in fund raising should also be made available to requesting institutions for consulting purposes.

It is strongly hoped that the various interest groups in allied health education will put aside their differences in order to advocate the continuation of funding programs on which future development depends. These groups include representatives of professional associations as well as educational institutions. Much of the special project activity recommended by the commission should involve joint effort of these groups; they should form more alliances for raising special project funds, for advocating their shared goals and objectives before federal and state legislative and regulatory bodies, and for assuring the future of allied health education and services.

Continuation and expansion of the necessary support for allied health education and services are most likely to be achieved if the broad allied health constituency communicates its needs effectively to planners and legislators. In many cases, this will require single presentations by professional associations or educators representing a segment of the educational arena, such as two-year colleges. Such efforts are particularly relevant when dealing with specific issues. However, when dealing with issues of broad concern, it is essential to present to legislative and regulatory bodies a consensus representing as large a constituency as possible, based on viewpoints of more than a single segment of allied health education and services.

The commission believes that ASAHP, as the only national organization representing the broad allied health constituency, including both educational institutions and professional groups, should strengthen its advocacy role in presenting matters of general concern to Congress and other national policymaking bodies. Its state chapters should assume leadership in advocating support for allied health education at state and local levels.

15.9: *ASAHP and its state chapters should educate health policy planners and legislators on the contribu-*

tions made by allied health personnel in order to promote necessary and appropriate support for continuation and expansion of allied health education and services.

Alliances for Education: Impact on Health

The recommendations of this commission are directed toward allied health education, but the impact of the recommendations should extend well beyond education and lead ultimately to improved health in the United States. Allied health practitioners constitute a major and increasingly vital segment of the health workforce. The occupations are young, growing, and well suited to the new challenges for health care delivery in the coming decades: to provide good health care to people in urban and rural areas that currently are medically underserved; to serve the special needs of the handicapped, the aged, and persons of various social and ethnic backgrounds; to better integrate physical and mental health services; to promote healthy life-styles and environments and prevent disability and disease; and to practice with an overriding concern for patients and clients as human beings and an appreciation of cost and quality control. The most direct way to accomplish these goals is to educate those who will provide these services and those who will assume leadership in improving their cost-effectiveness. The commission has recommended the formation of various kinds of alliances that link education closely to health service.

In an increasingly complex health delivery system, effective service depends on collaboration and an appreciation of the interdependence of health occupations. The commission has emphasized the value of the allied health concept as one that refers to "all health personnel working toward the common goal of providing the best possible services in patient care and health promotion." Specific collaborative activities among occupational groups are recommended here to achieve this alliance in practice. In particular, identification of commonalities in roles, functions, and knowledge base has great potential implications for both education and practice.

Many commission recommendations involve the forging

of alliances between educational institutions and professional groups. They should work together toward an allied health education that is linked to performance objectives based on a clear understanding of roles and functions of occupations, as well as changes in health services and delivery patterns. They should work together to increase complementarity and continuity among the four major components of allied health education: basic occupational preparation, on-the-job training, advanced education, and continuing education. They should adopt mechanisms to permit effective development of human resources in allied health fields and to encourage greater participation of disadvantaged minorities and women, particularly in leadership roles. They should collaborate to test and continually improve the methods of clinical practice, with an emphasis on quality and cost-effectiveness of such methods.

Alliances are recommended between educational institutions and clinical settings, as providers of clinical education and as employers. Closer integration of clinical and didactic education is seen as a major step toward making education responsive to practice needs, and increasing the range of clinical experiences is suggested to better prepare students to adapt to changing health care settings and services. Alliances between educational institutions and employers are recommended to ensure that programs are established, maintained, or terminated according to the demands of their service area.

Alliances between and within educational institutions also are proposed as a means of meeting educational goals that have direct implications for health service. Collaboration between institutions can have a particularly direct impact on health care by providing the necessary manpower to underserved areas. Moreover, interdisciplinary approaches to education can promote mutual understanding and colleagueship among allied health personnel as well as between allied health personnel and nurses, physicians, dentists, and others. Such colleagueship is essential for effective utilization of personnel and team practice.

Finally, the future of allied health education and the promise it holds for improved health in the United States will be determined by the extent to which alliances can be formed between educational institutions, occupational groups, and the various funding and regulatory boards. Allied health services depend on allied health education, and allied health education depends on the ability of the many individual interest groups to communicate the significance of these services actively and forcefully.

It is hoped that the work of the National Commission on Allied Health Education will not end with the publication of these findings and recommendations but rather will serve to generate initiative and action to achieve the goals of the future. The last decade was characterized by rapid growth and experimentation. The next decade will require a consolidation of efforts, weeding out the extravagant and redundant, more rational decision making, and improved utilization of resources. Most importantly, the next decade will demand a strong research commitment from allied health, courage to face and learn from efforts of the past, willingness to continue with innovation, and renewed determination to forge genuine alliances.

Appendix A

Methodology

Staff Analyses of Existing Data

The major existing data sources for this study were the inventories of educational programs for the 152 occupations listed in the *Glossary of Health Occupation Titles* that were conducted in 1973 and 1975 by the American Society of Allied Health Professions (ASAHP) and the American Hospital Association (AHA). These inventories used a comparable format and provided detailed descriptive information on the following numbers of occupational programs:

	ASAHP Inventories: Occupational Programs in Junior and Senior Colleges	*AHA Inventories: Occupational Programs in Hospitals*
1973	5,053	4,013
1975	5,584	4,273

The ASAHP records are estimated to contain information on about 75 percent of the universe of collegiate programs in the United States that offer basic occupational preparation, advanced education or training, and teacher training programs for these 152 occupations. The AHA records may contain information on as many as 90 percent of the "independently administered" hospital programs in the United States that provide either basic or advanced preparation for these same occupations.

Analyses of data on collegiate and hospital programs were supplemented by secondary analyses of data collected by the U.S. Office of Education (USOE) in its 1975 and 1977 Postsecondary Career School Surveys. The USOE surveys provided basic information on programs in enrollments in almost 100 percent of vocational education programs in noncollegiate postsecondary institutions such as public, private nonprofit, and proprietary vocational-technical and allied health career schools.

Survey of Professional Associations

Through an examination of documents, coupled with a postcard mailing to various associations, the staff identified 125 professional membership associations that represent occupations listed in the *Glossary of Health Occupation Titles.* Before mailing the survey questionnaire, the staff made telephone calls to each association, generally to the executive director or president, to explain the purpose of the survey and enlist cooperation. After a series of follow-up efforts, completed questionnaires were received in October 1978 from 79 associations, a 63 percent return rate. The responding associations represent 86 different allied health occupations.

The high response rate is remarkable in view of the length of the questionnaire and the time involved in providing information on all of the following topic areas:

- the association's membership and activities
- the occupations or specialties represented by the association (when established, number employed, credentialing, supervisory and career change patterns)
- current, future, and most appropriate educational settings for basic occupational preparation
- degree levels of personnel and relation of degree level to quality of work performance

- appropriateness and type of advanced training
- relation of education to practice needs and quality assurance mechanisms
- contributions to the body of knowledge in the field and scholarly activity
- leadership development (educational experiences that contributed to the development of teachers, administrators, managers, researchers, and advanced clinicians)
- practices, policies, and opinions regarding continuing education
- the meaning and value of the term *allied health*
- collaboration with other organizations
- perceived commonalities between occupations represented by the association and other health occupations

The serious attention given to the questionnaire is an indicator of the strong interest of professional associations in contributing to the future development of allied health education. In many cases, group effort was involved. Some questionnaires were filled out by several different individuals, with the president, executive director, and director of education or research each answering different types of questions. Some questionnaires were reviewed and discussed by advisory boards or by leaders gathered for the association's annual meeting.

Survey of Leaders

The staff undertook a survey of allied health leaders to identify career paths and patterns of leadership development, with particular attention to three question areas:

- What are the backgrounds—family, educational, and occupational—of allied health leaders?
- What strengths do they manifest?
- What are the career growth options in allied health?

To identify the survey population, the following steps were taken. First, the professional associations participating in the commission survey described earlier, as well as the two-year college program directors listed in the ASAHP membership directory, were asked for their nominations. Second, the names of deans and directors of allied health or related programs in four-year colleges and universities were compiled from a number of sources. Finally, the staff obtained the names of Kellogg Fellows and of allied health administrators who had participated in the Institute for College and University Administrators (ICUA) run by the American Council on Education's Office of Leadership Development in Higher Education; the purpose here was to determine whether participation in such training programs had an impact on careers.

A total of 364 questionnaires was sent out; exactly one half of the recipients responded. Response rates varied from two thirds of those in four-year colleges and universities to just one fourth of Kellogg Fellows. The low response rate of the last group is probably attributable to our having had only old addresses for these people. Respondents included 73 clinical leaders nominated by professional associations, 67 allied health administrators in four-year colleges and universities, 13 two-year college nominees, and 29 past participants in fellowship programs.

Informal Surveys of Allied Health Administrators. A major emphasis of the 1967 subcommittee report was the need for organizing allied health education programs in coordinated units where, it was thought, greater potential existed for resource sharing and exchange and for fostering the team approach to health care. The growth of allied health units between the 1967 report and the current study took place primarily in academic health centers. Currently, there are peer schools of allied health or health-related professions on at least 38 of the 122 medical school campuses in the United States, and an additional 22 medical schools have an allied health department or division. Although a definitive study of the effectiveness of such units was beyond the scope of this commission, a panel of allied health administrators in 23 academic health centers was utilized to shed some light on questions such as: What is the organizational structure for the administration of the allied health programs on these campuses? What is the status of allied health relative to other disciplines on these campuses? How much collaboration and research activity does the medical school environment foster? What are the advantages and disadvantages of different organizational arrangements? A first request, for information on organizational structure, programs, and funding, elicited responses from all 23 panelists. A second request, involving opinions and assessments, elicited responses from 13. In addition, the panelists were particularly helpful, when called upon as individuals, in providing information on innovative approaches and as a sounding board for findings and conclusions on various matters.

Other Informal Surveys. In addition, informal surveys were used to obtain information on specific topics. To learn more about the involvement of allied health programs in consortium arrangements, letters were sent to postsecondary education agencies (for collegiate and vocational-technical education) in all fifty states, as well as known consortia. To explore the impact of federal funding, a telephone survey was conducted with administrators whose project funds had not been renewed. To understand some of the factors involved in terminating allied health programs, a telephone survey was conducted with high-level administrators in institutions that reported particular programs in 1973 but not in 1975. This type of information gathering, which can be described as investigative reporting, was used on a lesser scale to shed light on numerous questions that arose during the documentation stage.

Assessment of Recommendations

A first set of recommendations was developed by the three commission task forces at meetings in February and April of 1979 and sent to all the commissioners for review. From their assessment of each recommendation, it was possible to identify those that were considered of high and low priority, as well as major areas of disagreement. The three task force leaders, Donald W. Fisher, Jack H. Hall, and Dorothy McMullan, met subsequently with Chairman Dickey and the staff to discuss the results of the assessment and plan for the June meeting of the commission. Most of the recommendations that appear in this report were discussed, revised, and agreed upon by the full commission at the June 1979 meeting.

All the recommendations selected by the commissioners are considered important for guiding allied health education in the future, but not all can be expected to have equal impact. In order to identify the key recommendations that are listed in the summary, the commissioners were asked to rate a list of recommendations on four criteria:

- impact on patient care and/or community health
- impact on educational institutions
- impact on students
- feasibility

These criteria reflect the basic concerns of the commissioners for the quality of allied health education and health services in the United States and for fairness to the student. Based on the results of this rating, and a full commission discussion on September 8, 1979, the commissioners selected fifteen recommendations as crucial to allied health education and services in the next decade.

Appendix B

ASAHP *Glossary*

1975 Inventory of Health Occupations Education Programs in Two-Year and Four-Year Colleges and Universities: Major Category Inclusions

01 Administration, Planning, and Office
03 Biomedical Engineering
05 Clinical Laboratory Services
07 Dental Services
10 Dietetic and Nutrition Services
13 Emergency Services
16 Environmental Services
19 Health Education
95 Health Professionals Not Elsewhere Classified
22 Health-Related Teacher Preparation
25 Information and Communication
34 Medical Instrumentation and Machine Operation
37 Medical Record
40 Mental Health
42 Nuclear Medicine
43 Nursing-Related Services
49 Pharmacy Services
58 Physician Extender
61 Podiatric Services
67 Radiological Services
70 Rehabilitation-Occupational
73 Rehabilitation-Physical

76 Rehabilitation Not Elsewhere Classified
80 Respiratory Therapy Services
85 Social Services and Counseling
88 Speech and Hearing Services
91 Veterinary Services
46 Vision Care

Glossary of Occupational Titles

01 **Administration, Planning, and Office personnel function at various levels to maintain and operate clinical offices and institutions and to plan for improved health care and delivery.**

0105 Health Economist: Applies specialized knowledge of the laws of supply and demand, marketing, polling, econometrics, and motivation research to permit the efficient delivery of health services.

0110 Health Care Administrator: Occupies top-level positions in a variety of health care settings: hospitals, official health agencies, long-term care facilities, social service agencies, voluntary and tax-paying health agencies, and public health agencies. Policy development, activity coordination, procedural development, and planning are the primary functions of the position.

0115 Health Care Assistant Administrator: Occupies middle management positions in a variety of clinical and health care settings: hospitals, public and private health agencies, long-term care facilities, social service agencies.

0120 Health Planner: Works in state and areawide health planning agencies and related programs implementing community goals, including planning and evaluating developmental policies.

0125 Health Systems Analyst: Develops and applies the principles of industrial and systems engineering, operations research, and management to the design, evaluation, and implementation of improved health care.

0136 Long-Term Care Administrator: Directs and coordinates all operations and activities of extended care facilities.

0140 Medical/Dental Secretary: Assists physicians and/or dentists through the use of medical shorthand, typing, filing, accounting, appointment scheduling, receptionist duties, and office management.

0145 Medical Office Assistant: Assumes responsibility for routine administrative, clerical, and record-keeping procedures in a physician's office, assists the physician in medical examinations and treatments, and cares for medical equipment and supplies.

0150 Rehabilitation Administrator: Manages a rehabilitation agency's business aspects: personnel, budget control, public relations work, training, programs planning, and services coordination.

0155 Unit Clerk: Handles routine clerical and reception work in a floor nursing unit: receiving patients and visitors, scheduling appointments, monitoring the location of all ward staff, and, where hospital policy permits, transcribing doctors' orders, ordering supplies, and updating information on patients' charts. (Ward Clerk)

0156 Unit Manager: Supervises and coordinates administrative management functions for one or more patient care units: oversees unit clerks, initiates clerical procedures and serves as a liaison for the unit with other hospital departments. (Ward Service Manager, Ward Supervisor)

03 Biomedical Engineering personnel combine basic engineering and biomedical science in order to design, assemble, and adapt medical devices, instruments, and processes to improve the quality and cost in the delivery of medical health care.

0305 Biomedical Engineer: Utilizes engineering ideas and techniques in the development of new instruments, equipment, processes, and systems for the medical care of patients and the improvement of health systems.

0310 Biomedical Engineering Technician: Assembles, repairs, and adapts medical equipment to assist biomedical engineers, physicians, and scientists in the development and maintenance of medical equipment and systems for the delivery of medical and health care. (Biomedical Equipment Technician)

05 Clinical Laboratory Services personnel work in a clinical laboratory setting, collecting, mounting, processing, classifying and analyzing laboratory specimens.

0505 Specialist in Blood Bank Technology: Medical technologist, working under the direction of a pathologist, physician, or laboratory director, is prepared to collect, classify, store, and process blood, including preparation of components from whole blood, detection and identification of antibodies in patient and donor bloods, and selection and delivery of suitable blood for transfusion.

0510 Chemistry Technologist: Works under the supervision of a pathologist, physician, or qualified scientist in performing qualitative and quantitative chemical analyses of body fluids and exudates, utilizing quantitative equipment and a wide range of laboratory instruments, to provide information for diagnosing and treating diseases.

0515 Cytotechnologist: Works under the supervision of a pathologist, physician, or medical technologist in handling, staining, mounting, and evaluating cells from the human body to determine cellular variations and abnormalities such as cancer and other physiologic changes.

0519 Hematologist: Directs and supervises analysis and testing of blood specimens, and interprets test results toward disease treatment. Directs operations of hospital blood bank, which involves supervision of hematology technologists and blood bank technologists, and develops diagnostic reports for approval by the pathologist.

0520 Hematology Technologist: Works under supervision of a hematologist, medical technologist, or laboratory director in performing quantitative, qualitative, and coagulation tests on cellular and plasma components of blood for use in the diagnosis and treatment of disease.

0525 Histologic Technician: Works under supervision of a pathologist or other qualified physician in sectioning, staining, and mounting human or animal tissues and fluid for microscopic study.

0530 Medical Laboratory Assistant: Works under the direct supervision of a medical technologist, pathologist, physician, or qualified scientist in performing routine laboratory procedures requiring basic technical skills and minimal independent judgment, in chemistry, hematology, and microbiology. (Certified Laboratory Assistant)

0535 Medical Laboratory Scientist: Performs clinical analysis procedures and research in the medical/clinical laboratories utilizing disciplines such as chemistry, biochemistry, bacteriology, and microbiology.

0540 Medical Laboratory Technician: Works under the supervision of a medical technologist, pathologist, or physician in performing more complex or specialized bacteriological, biological, and chemical tests requiring limited independent judgment or correlation competency, to provide data for use in the diagnosis and evaluation of effective treatment of disease.

0545 Medical Technologist: Performs a wide range of complex and specialized procedures in all general areas of the clinical laboratory, making independent and correlation judgments and working in conjunction with pathologists, physicians, and qualified scientists. May supervise and/or teach laboratory personnel.

0550 Microbiology Technologist: Works with a minimum of supervision by a pathologist, physician, or laboratory director in performing many bacteriological, viral, parasitological, immunologic, and serologic procedures in a clinical laboratory setting.

0555 Public Health Laboratory Scientist: Performs clinical laboratory procedures and research with specific public health focus or within a public health setting.

0560 Prosector: Performs complete gross autopsies under the supervision of a physician, cuts blocks for slides, applies special stains for bacteria, and freezes sections for rapid diagnosis.

07 Dental Services personnel render varieties of services to the dentist; they do general office work, laboratory work, and they assist the dentist at the chairside.

0720 Dental Assistant: Assists dentist at the chairside in dental operatory, performs reception and clerical functions, and carries out dental radiography and selected dental laboratory work.

0725 Dental Hygienists: Are professional oral health clinicians and educators who help the public develop and maintain optimum oral health. As members of the dental health team, dental hygienists perform preventive, restorative, and therapeutic services under the supervision of a dentist. Dental hygienists are the only licensed dental auxiliary and specific responsibilities vary, depending on the state dental practice act.

0730 Dental Technician: Is prepared to construct complete and partial dentures, make orthodontic appliances, fix bridgework, crowns, and other dental restorations and appliances, as authorized by dentists. (Dental Laboratory Technician)

10 **Dietetic and Nutrition Services personnel translate nutritional needs into the selection, purchasing, preparation, and service of appropriate foods, along with maintenance of equipment, sanitation, and cost control. They provide nutritional education to individuals and groups and serve as nutritional consultants to health facilities and communities.**

1005 Dietary Aide: Performs nontechnical food preparation routines, as directed by a supervisor, serves meals to patients, and assists with food-related jobs in health care facilities. (Dietetic Aide)

1010 Dietetic Technician: Functions as middle management and service personnel in the nutritional care of individuals in health care facilities, assisting with the planning, implementation, and evaluation of food programs, working with both the food service supervisor and the dietitian and, where hospital policy permits, may train and supervise dietary aides. (Food Service Manager, Food Service Assistant, Food Service Technician)

1015 Dietitian: Applies the principles of nutrition and management in administering institutional food service programs, plans special diets at physicians' requests, and instructs individuals and groups in the application of nutrition principles to the selection of food.

1020 Dietitian/Nutritionist: Trained in dietetics and/or nutrition.

1025 Dietetic Assistant: Writes food menus following dietetic specifications, coordinates food service to patients, orders supplies, maintains sanitation, and oversees the work of food service employees in health care facilities. (Food Service Supervisor)

1030 Nutritionist: Adapts and applies food and nutrient information to the solution of food problems, the control of disease, and the promotion of health, performs nutrition research, instructs groups and individuals about nutritional requirements, and helps people develop meal patterns to meet their nutritional needs.

13 **Emergency Services personnel administer temporary medical help by responding to, evaluating, and assisting in emergency conditions.**

1305 Ambulance Attendant: Provides first aid and assistance in the transportation of critically ill and injured persons.

1310 Emergency and/or Disaster Specialist: Develops and implements hospitalwide procedures for dealing with in-house and community emergencies and disasters.

1315 Emergency Medical Technician: Responds to medical emergency calls, evaluates the nature of the emergency, and carries out specified diagnostic and emergency treatment procedures under standing orders or the specific directions of a physician.

16 **Environmental Services personnel inspect, evaluate, and gather data for their use in the design, operation, and control of systems for prevention and elimination of environmental hazards.**

1605 Environmental Engineer: Applies engineering principles to the control, elimination, and prevention of environmental hazards such as air pollution, water pollution, solids pollution, and noise pollution. (Sanitary Engineer)

1610 Environmental Engineering Assistant: Works with and assists the environmental engineer in his tasks of designing and controlling systems to eliminate and control environmental health hazards.

1615 Environmental Health Technician: Assists in the survey of environmental hazards and performs technical duties under professional supervision in many areas of environmental health such as pollution control, radiation protection, and sanitation protection. (Sanitarian Technician)

1620 Environmentalist: Plans, develops, and implements standards and systems to improve the quality of air, water, food, shelter, and other environmental factors, manages comprehensive environmental health programs, and promotes public awareness of the need to prevent and eliminate environmental health hazards. (Sanitarian)

1623 Health Care Facilities Housekeeper: Develops, implements, and supervises techniques used to control, eliminate, and prevent cross infection or other environmental hazards in health care facilities. Establishes standards and work procedures for the housekeeping staff in accordance with the established policies of the facility. Maintains budgets, inventories of supplies and equipment, and personnel hiring practices.

1625 Industrial Hygienist: Conducts programs in industry to measure and to help control, eliminate, and prevent occupational hazards and diseases.

1630 Sanitarian Aide: Collects and measures environmental sanitation conditions and implements corrective action on health hazards for which specific guidelines exist.

19 **Health Education personnel acquaint groups and individuals with the standards of optimum health and the principles of achieving and maintaining optimum health.**

1905 Community/Public Health Educator: Alerts community groups and individuals to changing patterns of health care, to health hazards, and to activities that will promote community health and safety.

1910 School Health Educator: Teaches elementary,

secondary, and college students principles of personal health sciences, total fitness, family living, consumer and environmental health, and community health trends and resources.

1915 Health Educator: Influences public attitudes toward achieving and maintaining high standards of health care through teaching and utilizing school and community resources, as well as providing consultation to school administrators, health councils, and community groups.

95 Health Professionals Not Elsewhere Classified

9505 Biostatistician: Uses statistical theory, techniques, and methods to determine useful measurements or meaningful relationships of information relating to health or disease.

9510 Epidemiologist: Is concerned with determining the distribution and causal factors of health problems, encompassing areas such as acute and chronic illness, communicable diseases, behavioral disorders, alcoholism, and drug abuse.

9515 Health Physicist: Directs research, training, and monitoring programs to protect hospital patients and laboratory personnel from radiation hazards, inspects and evaluates standards and decontamination procedures, and develops new methods to safeguard humans and their environment against unnecessary radiation exposure.

9520 Health Physics Technician: Monitors radiation levels, gives instructions in radiation safety, labels radioactive materials, and assists the health physicist in conducting experimental studies in radiation.

9525 Population and Family Planning Specialist: Uses demography, demographic techniques, and reproductive physiology to plan, conduct, and evaluate family planning programs.

9530 Public Health Practitioner—Not Elsewhere Classified: Professionally trained to work in a public health capacity not specifically defined elsewhere in this *Glossary*.

9535 Toxicologist: Is concerned with the nature and extent of the injurious response to the ingestion of chemical compounds and the determination of safe levels of exposure or ingestion in man and other species.

9536 Vocational Evaluator: Assesses needs of those with employment handicaps as a result of physical, mental, or emotional disability. Evaluates work behavior and vocational potential by collecting and/or administering and interpreting relevant biographical data, task data, work samples, psychometrics, and situational assessments, and interprets findings to the rehabilitation counselor.

22 **Health-Related Teacher Preparation combines teaching skills and health expertise in preparing: (1) instructors of individuals who are physically disabled, emotionally disturbed, or mentally retarded; and (2) allied health professionals who desire to teach within their specialty area.**

2205 Allied Health Educator: Teaches the specialty in which he or she was trained to students being prepared in the discipline. May also supervise other individuals in his or her occupation.

2210 Teacher of the Deaf: Adapts methods and curricula in the teaching of special skills, elementary, and secondary school subjects to deaf and hard-of-hearing pupils.

2215 Teacher of the Emotionally Disturbed: Conducts educational programs for emotionally disturbed pupils.

2220 Teacher of the Learning Disabled: Develops and implements educational programs to assist children in overcoming or compensating for learning disabilities such as aphasia, dyslexia, or other related problems.

2225 Teacher of the Mentally Retarded: Develops and implements educational programs for trainable or educable mentally retarded persons according to the pupil's level of learning.

2230 Teacher of the Physically Handicapped: Develops and implements academic and recreational programs for handicapped persons after evaluating the physical limitations, abilities, and needs of the individuals.

2232 Teacher of Special Education—Not Elsewhere Classified: Develops and implements educational programs suited to the needs of students with physical disabilities, mental retardation, or emotional disturbances.

2235 Teacher of the Visually Handicapped: Teaches academic and practical skills to the blind or visually handicapped through the use of braille and other specialized methods.

25 **Information and Communication personnel apply a communications orientation to the development, presentation, organization, and recording of medical facts and material for the benefit of medical personnel and the general public.**

2505 Health Writer: Specializes in the writing of health or medical materials.

2510 Medical Communications Specialist: Knows the properties and capabilities of communications media and applies this knowledge to the design and improvement of communication processes in the health field.

2515 Medical Computer Specialist: Combines a knowledge of computer science and health science to provide systems and programming support in the medical field.

2520 Medical Illustrator: Demonstrates medical facts by the creation of illustrations, models, and teaching films; serves as a consultant, advisor, and administrator in the field of medical illustration.

2525 Medical Librarian: Combines a degree in library science with specialized knowledge of medical librarianship and bibliography to acquire, organize, catalogue, retrieve, and disseminate medical information.

2530 Medical Library Assistant: Combines training in library technology and health subjects to assist medical librarians in the process of acquiring, organizing, cataloguing, retrieving, and disseminating medical information.

2535 Medical Photographer: Visually presents medical facts by means of lantern slides, motion pictures, photographs of patients, reproduction of x-rays, and/or photomicrographs.

34 **Medical Instrumentation and Machine Operation personnel maintain and/or operate equipment and instruments that**

supplement and support body functions or that provide diagnostic or therapeutic services.

3405 Cardiopulmonary Technician: Performs a wide range of tests related to the functions and therapeutic care of the heart-lung system, operates and maintains a heart-lung machine for extracorporeal circulation, assists in cardiac catheterization and cardiac resuscitation, and assists in the postoperative monitoring, care, and treatment of heart-lung patients.

3412 Circulation Technologist: Operates and designs heart-lung machines, dialysis machines, artificial organs, and similar circulation devices and monitoring instruments to provide circulatory support to patients.

3415 Dialysis Technician: Operates and maintains an artificial kidney machine following approved methods and techniques to provide dialysis treatment for patients with kidney disorders or failures.

3420 Electrocardiographic Technician: Operates and maintains electrocardiograph machines, records electromotive variation in heart muscle action, and provides data for diagnosis and treatment of heart ailments by physicians.

3425 Electroencephalographic/Electrocardiographic Technician: Operates and maintains electroencephalographic and electrocardiographic machines.

3430 Electroencephalographic Technologist/Technician: Operates and maintains electroencephalographic machines, recording brain waves on a graph to be used by physicians in the diagnosis of brain disorders.

3435 Electromyographic Technician: Assists physicians in recording and analyzing bioelectric potentials that originate in muscle tissue, including the operation of various electronic devices, maintenance of electronic equipment, assisting with patient care, and record keeping.

37 **Medical Record personnel plan, organize, and manage patient information systems and statistical reports for medical and administrative staff use and health care research.**

3705 Medical Record Administrator: Plans, designs, develops, and manages systems of patient information, administrative and clinical statistical data, and patient medical records, in all types of health care institutions.

3710 Medical Record Technician: Serves as the skilled assistant to the medical record administrator, carrying out the technical work of coding, analyzing, and preserving patients' medical records and compiling reports, disease indices, and statistics in health care institutions.

3715 Medical Transcriptionist: Is skilled in typing, medical spelling, medical terminology, and the proper format of medical records and reports; is prepared to transcribe medical dictation using mechanical dictating equipment.

40 Mental Health personnel assist the health professionals in the prevention and treatment of mental disorders through recreational, occupational, and educational programs.

4002 Human Services Technologist/Technician: Employs skills as a generalist, based upon knowledge of human behavior and social problems in settings providing mental health and social rehabilitation services; employs a whole person, noncustodial approach to treating the symptomatic and causative elements that affect the individual's ability to respond to the social environment.

4005 Mental Health Associate/Technician/Assistant: Works under the supervision of professional personnel in supplementing physical care for persons with emotional problems through recreational, occupational, and readjustment activities, including participation in group therapy with clients and families; refers patients to community agencies, and visits patients after their release from an institution.

4010 Mental Health Technologist: Works with other mental health professionals in diagnosing psychiatric disorders, counseling, and planning treatment for the emotionally disturbed or mentally retarded.

4015 Mental Retardation Aide: Works under the supervision of a professional staff in attending to the physical needs and well-being of mentally retarded patients and in assisting with teaching and recreation processes.

4020 Psychiatric Technician: Works under the supervision of professional and/or technical personnel in caring for mentally ill patients in a psychiatric medical care facility; assists in carrying out the prescribed treatment plan for the patient; maintains consistent attitudes in communicating with the patient in keeping with the treatment plan, and carries out assigned individual and group activities with patients. (Psychiatric Aide)

42 **Nuclear Medicine personnel prepare or use radioactive nuclides in laboratory procedures, scanning-imaging, and function studies for diagnostic, therapeutic, and research purposes.**

4205 Nuclear Medicine Technologist/Technician: Performs a wide variety of diagnostic tests in human beings and/or on body fluids utilizing radioactivity and/or stable nuclides. Also applies radioactivity in the course of treatment. Makes independent judgments under the general guidance of a nuclear medicine physician.

43 **Nursing-Related Services personnel assist the physician in bedside patient care and provide specialty services as required by institutional and community needs.**

4342 Nurse Aide/Orderly: Performs tasks delegated or assigned by the professional nursing staff, including assisting in providing direct patient care of a routine nature, making beds, delivering messages, counting linens, and escorting patients to other departments in the hospital. May also include, where hospital policy permits, the taking of vital signs, and in the case of orderlies, includes performing heavier work in the nursing unit and maintaining equipment and may include setting up of traction and performing male catheterization. (Nurse Assistant, Nurse Aide, Orderly, Hospital Attendant, Nurse Attendant)

4345 Nurse Anesthetist: Registered nurse prepared to work under an anesthesiologist or physician in administering anesthetic agents to patients before and after surgical and obstetrical operations and other medical procedures.

4350 Nurse-Midwife: Assumes responsibility for the

care of apparently normal obstetrical patients during pregnancy, labor, delivery, and postnatal period.

4355 Nurse Practitioner: Registered nurse prepared to carry out functions previously performed by the general practitioner or physician specialist; collaborates with other health professionals in planning and instituting programs for the delivery of primary, acute, or chronic care; provides direct care to clients by making independent decisions about nursing care needs.

4360 Obstetrical Technician: Assists in the care of mothers in labor and delivery rooms before, during, and after delivery under supervision of professional personnel, including hygienic procedures, routine laboratory work, and sterilization of equipment and supplies.

4365 Operating Room Technician: Works as general technical assistant on the surgical team by arranging supplies and instruments in the operating room, maintaining antiseptic conditions, preparing patients for surgery and assisting the surgeon during the operation.

4371 Geriatric Care Worker: Administers to the needs of aged patients, bringing to the task an understanding of the problems of institutionalization, economic needs, and attitudes toward the elderly as these concepts relate to this specific population.

49 **Pharmacy Services personnel assist the pharmacist in selected activities in pharmacy departments to provide pharmaceutical services to patients, nurses, and physicians.**

4919 Medication Pharmacy Technician: Works under the supervision of a pharmacist; administers drugs to patients except for intravenous medications.

4920 Pharmacy Technician: Assists the pharmacist in selected activities including medication profile reviews for drug incompatibilities, typing prescription labels, prescription packaging, handling of purchase records, inventory control, and may, where hospital policy and state law permit, administer drugs to patients under the supervision of a registered pharmacist.

58 **Physician Extender personnel render direct and specific assistance to the physician specialist and general practitioner in clinical and research endeavors, taking medical histories, performing detailed physical examinations, and conducting visual, auditory, developmental, and laboratory tests.**

5805 Physician Assistant-Primary Care: Performs physician-delegated functions in the areas of general practice, including family medicine, internal medicine, pediatrics, obstetrics, and emergency medicine.

5810 Physician Assistant-Specialty: Performs functions delegated by a clinical specialist in specific areas of patient care: urology, surgery, pathology, orthopedics, etc.

61 **Podiatric Services personnel work under the direct supervision of the podiatrist, performing supplementary duties for the foot specialist.**

6120 Podiatric Assistant: Supports the podiatrist in his service to patients by preparing patients for treatment, sterilizing the instruments, performing general office duties, and assisting the podiatrist in preparing dressings, administering treatments, and developing x-rays.

67 **Radiological Services personnel use ionizing radiation for diagnostic, therapeutic, and research purposes.**

6705 Medical Radiation Dosimetrist: Calculates radiation dosage in the treatment of malignant disease and plans the direction of radiation to its target in the safest way.

6710 Radiation Therapy Technologist/Technician: Administers x-rays and electron beam equipment in order to treat disease in patients and assists in preparing and handling radioactive materials for therapy purposes.

6715 Radiologic Technologist/Technician: Maintains and safely uses equipment and supplies necessary to demonstrate portions of the human body on x-ray film or fluoroscopic screen for diagnostic purposes. May supervise and/or teach radiologic personnel. (X-Ray Technician)

6720 Ultrasound Technical Specialist: Uses acoustic energy for diagnosis, research, and therapy, operates ultrasound equipment to obtain diagnostic results, evaluates results for quality of technique, and, in emergency situations, makes interim reports to medical staff.

70 **Rehabilitation-Occupational personnel use work-related skills in treating or training patients who are physically or mentally ill, in preventing disability, in evaluating behavior, and in restoring disabled persons to health, social, or economic independence.**

7005 Manual Arts Therapist: Uses industrial arts, workshops, and agricultural activities to assist in the rehabilitation of patients.

7010 Occupational Therapist: Evaluates the self care, work, and play/leisure time task performance skills of well and disabled clients of all age ranges; plans and implements programs, social and interpersonal activities designed to restore, develop and/or maintain the client's ability to accomplish satisfactorily those daily living tasks required of his or her specific age and necessary to his or her particular occupational role adjustment.

7015 Occupational Therapy Assistant: Works under the supervision of an occupational therapist in evaluating clients, planning and implementing programs designed to restore or develop a client's self care, work, and play/leisure time task performance skills. Although the assistant requires supervision in conducting a remedial program, he or she can function independently when conducting a maintenance program.

7020 Rehabilitation Homemaking Specialist: Trains disabled homemakers to perform normal household activities in spite of their disability.

73 **Rehabilitation-Physical personnel use physical agents, assistive devices, and therapeutic exercise for the prevention of disease and disability and toward restoration of function to disabled persons.**

7305 Corrective Therapist/Adapted Physical Education Director: Provides medically prescribed programs of therapeutic exercise to physically and mentally ill patients to prevent muscular deconditioning resulting from inactivity and to attain resocialization and specific psychiatric objectives.

7310 Exercise Physiologist: Works with clinicians in hospitals with rehabilitation programs to provide exercise stress testing and cardiovascular rehabilitation for patients.

7312 Orthopedic Technician: Sets up traction rooms, applies all types of traction, makes casts, applies splints, and may train patients to operate a circle-o-bed.

7315 Orthotic/Prosthetic Assistant: Assists the orthotist/prosthetist in caring for patients by making casts, measurements, and model specifications and fitting supportive appliances and/or artificial limbs.

7320 Orthotic/Prosthetic Technician: Fabricates and repairs supportive appliances and/or artificial limbs under the guidance of the orthotist/prosthetist and his or her assistant.

7325 Orthotist/Prosthetist: Writes specifications for, makes, fits, and repairs braces and appliances and/or artificial limbs following the prescription of physicians.

7330 Physical Therapist: Uses physical agents, biomechanical and neurophysiological principles, and assistive devices in relieving pain, restoring maximum function, and preventing disability following disease, injury, or loss of bodily part.

7335 Physical Therapy Assistant: Assists the physical therapist by assembling equipment, carrying out specified treatment programs, and helping with complex treatment procedures. Other duties include responsibility for the personal care of patients, safety precautions, routine clerical and maintenance work.

76 **Rehabilitation Not Elsewhere Classified personnel apply the principles of rehabilitation to diversified areas of therapeutic technique, such as education, fine arts, and recreation.**

7605 Art Therapist: Applies the principles and techniques of arts to the rehabilitation of physically and mentally ill patients.

7610 Dance Therapist: Applies the principles and techniques of dance to the rehabilitation of physically and mentally ill patients.

7615 Educational Therapist: Instructs patients in academic and vocational subjects to further their medical recovery and prevent mental deconditioning.

7620 Music Therapist: Uses individual and group musical activities with physically and mentally ill patients to accomplish therapeutic aims, to create an environment conducive to treatment, or to influence behavior.

7625 Recreational Therapist: Plans, organizes, and directs medically approved recreation programs such as sports, trips, dramatics, and arts and crafts, to help clients either in recovery from illness or in coping with temporary or permanent disability.

7630 Recreational Therapy Technician: Assists the recreational therapist in conducting medically approved recreation programs such as sports, trips, dramatics, and arts and crafts.

7635 Rehabilitation Therapy Assistant: Is prepared by a general orientation to various rehabilitation specialties to assist the professional therapist in carrying out rehabilitation programs.

80 **Respiratory Therapy Services personnel, under medical direction, treat, manage, control, and perform diagnostic evaluations in the care of patients with deficiencies and abnormalities in the cardio-pulmonary system.**

8040 Respiratory Therapist: Administers respiratory care under the direction of a physician, evaluating the patient's progress and making recommendations for respiratory therapy. His or her proficiencies include ventilatory therapy, cardio-respiratory rehabilitation, microenvironmental control, and diagnostic testing of the respiratory system. (Inhalation Therapist)

8045 Respiratory Therapy Technician: Routinely

treats patients requiring noncritical respiratory care and recognizes and responds to a limited number of specified patient respiratory emergencies.

85 **Social Services and Counseling personnel use individual or group counseling techniques and/or provide services offered by social agencies to assist individuals in personal and/or social adjustment.**

8505 Alcohol/Drug Abuse Specialist: Advises and assists people in their efforts to overcome personal, family, and social problems that are manifested in alcoholism and drug addiction.

8510 Clinical Pastoral Counselor: Combines a knowledge of health and religion in counseling the confined ill and disabled.

8515 Community Health Worker: Assists people in the community with medical, social, or mental health problems in finding and utilizing sources of available help.

8520 Genetic Assistant: Obtains complete genetic case histories from families of patients with inherited diseases and birth defects to be used in genetic counseling.

8525 Genetic Counselor: Counsels clients as to the origin, transmission, and development of hereditary characteristics and their relations to birth abnormalities.

8530 Homemaker/Home Health Aide: Assists with meals, shopping, household chores, bathing, and the other daily living needs, both physical and emotional, of elderly, ill, or disabled persons, working under professional supervision required by the situation.

8535 Medical Social Worker: Is prepared to identify and understand the social and emotional factors underlying patients' illness and to communicate these factors to the health team; to assist patients and their families in understanding and accepting the treatment necessary to maximize medical benefits and their adjustment to permanent and temporary effects of illness; and to utilize resources, such as family and community agencies, in assisting patients to recovery.

8536 Medical/Psychiatric Social Worker: Provides

the link between organized social services and those who need the services in order to solve social or medical problems. Through casework, groupwork, and community organization, assumes responsibility for aiding families and individuals with problems resulting from severe physical, mental, or emotional disabilities.

8540 Psychiatric Social Worker: Serves as a liaison between the psychiatrist, patient, and patient's family to provide counseling and emotional support to the patient and to contribute to the evaluation and diagnosis of mental disorders as a member of the psychiatric team.

8542 Rehabilitation Counselor: Helps disabled individuals become aware of and secure rehabilitation services designed to fit the disabled person for gainful employment; assists in job placement and checks on job satisfaction after employment.

8543 Rehabilitation Counselor Aide: Aids the rehabilitation counselor in developing and implementing a rehabilitation plan for an individual; under supervision, may conduct client interviews, locate and file data about employment opportunities, match clients with jobs available, and locate additional individuals in need of counseling or rehabilitation services.

8545 School Health Aide: Assists the physician or nurse with physical examinations and programs to improve or maintain students' health.

8546 Child Care Worker: Under supervision, implements activity and training programs that provide a preventive and therapeutic environment for mentally ill and emotionally disturbed children and adolescents. Trains children in self-help skills through intensive group sessions involving structured daily activities and reinforcement of other therapeutic experiences; records, evaluates, and reports progress of clients.

88 Speech and Hearing Services personnel evaluate, record, habilitate, and research speech and hearing disorders in children and adults.

8805 Audiologist: Evaluates hearing function and

performs research related to hearing; plans, directs, and conducts habilitative programs designed to improve the communication efficiency of individuals with impaired hearing.

8806 Audiologist (Pre-Master's): Qualified for entry into graduate-level training as an Audiologist.

8810 Speech/Hearing Therapy Aide: Assists in testing, evaluating, and treating the problems of people with speech and hearing difficulties.

8815 Speech Pathologist: Evaluates, habilitates, and performs research related to speech and language problems; plans, directs, and conducts remedial programs designed to restore or improve communication efficiency of individuals with language and speech impairments, whether arising from physiological neurological disturbances, defective articulation, or foreign dialect in children or adults.

8816 Speech Pathologist (Pre-Master's): In certain areas, treats speech and language disorders in children and adults and is prepared for graduate work in Speech Pathology.

8820 Speech Pathologist/Audiologist: Evaluates and habilitates hearing, speech, and language disorders, such as neurological disturbances, defective articulation, or foreign dialect in children or adults.

8821 Speech Pathologist/Audiologist (Pre-Master's): In certain areas, evaluates and treats speech and language disorders in children and adults and is prepared for graduate work in Speech Pathology or Audiology.

91 **Veterinary Services personnel work at the care, use, production, and husbandry of animals in a medical setting.**

9120 Laboratory Animal Specialist: Manages the husbandry, production, and use of laboratory animals including responsibility for the sanitation, caging, safety, and nutrition of animals and the business management of the animal laboratory.

9125 Laboratory Animal Worker: Cares for the health of laboratory animals used in research by feeding the animals, cleaning cages, preparing the animals for experiments, administering medications, and keeping records on laboratory procedures.

46 **Vision Care personnel work with or carry out the prescriptions of the ophthalmologist and optometrist. Their duties include ophthalmic examinations, treatment, and correction of ophthalmic disorders by physical or mechanical measures.**

4620 Ophthalmic Assistant/Technician: Assists the ophthalmologist in eye examinations and in the treatment of eye diseases and disorders.

4625 Ophthalmic Dispenser: Adapts and fits corrective eyewear as prescribed by the ophthalmologist or optometrist.

4630 Ophthalmic Laboratory Technician: Operates machines to grind lenses and fabricate eyewear to prescription.

4631 Ophthalmic Optician: Grinds lenses and fabricates eyewear, as well as adapts and fits corrective eyewear according to prescription by the opthalmologist or optometrist.

4635 Optometric Assistant/Technician: Assists an optometrist in diversified ways, including general office duties, vision testing patients, administering eye exercises, preparing and fitting corrective lenses, and styling eyewear.

4640 Orthoptist: Works under supervision of an ophthalmologist in testing for certain eye muscle imbalances and teaching the patient exercises to correct eye-coordination defects.

Appendix C

Carnegie Classification of Higher Education Institutions

To determine more precisely which kinds of higher education institutions have allied health programs, an updated version of the classification of higher education institutions developed by the Carnegie Commission on Higher Education in 1970 was utilized. This classification identifies five relatively homogeneous categories of colleges and universities and a number of subcategories based upon their functions as well as characteristics of their students and faculty. The Carnegie classification differs from the classification used by the U.S. Office of Education in that it treats each campus as an institution, whereas the Office of Education treats multicampus systems as single institutions.

An updated version of the Carnegie Classification for 1975-76 was provided by the American Council on Education.

In 1975-76, the Office of Education listed 3,056 institutions of higher education; because of the difference in treating multi-campus institutions, more institutions (3,092) were identified using the Carnegie Classification. These institutions were classified as follows:

1. *Doctoral-Granting Institutions.* Only 184 universities, just 6 percent of the nation's higher education institutions, are included in the broad category of doctoral-granting institutions. The category is further subdivided, based on the size of federal financial support received for academic sciences and on Ph.D. production, into four groups: Research Universities I and II and Doctoral-Granting Universities I and II. Research Universities I category includes the nation's most prestigious research universities, many with medical schools on their campuses, including 31 academic health centers. Doctoral-Granting Universities I and II have smaller numbers of doctoral programs, award fewer degrees, and receive less federal support than do Research Universities I and II.

2. *Comprehensive Universities and Colleges.* Comprehensive universities and colleges are much more numerous than doctoral-granting institutions and include about 597, or just under one fifth, of the nation's higher education institutions. Comprehensive Universities and Colleges I include institutions offering a liberal arts program and professional or occupational programs and enrolling at least 2,000 students. Some of these institutions award master's degrees. Some doctoral programs also are offered but represent a very minor portion of these institutions' educational activity. Comprehensive Universities and Colleges II category contains state colleges and some private colleges that offer a liberal arts program and at least one professional or occupational program, such as teacher training or nursing.

3. *Liberal Arts Colleges.* This group of colleges with a strong liberal arts tradition contains 600, or just under one fifth, of the nation's higher education institutions and has two subcategories, determined primarily on the basis of prestige of the institution and selectivity of its admission requirements. Liberal Arts Colleges I are among the nation's most selective baccalaureate-granting institutions. Their graduates are more

likely than others to continue study toward a Ph.D. at one of the leading doctoral institutions. Liberal Arts Colleges II include those not meeting the criteria for Category I; many are heavily involved in teacher training, although they grant degrees in arts and sciences rather than in education.

4. *Two-Year Colleges and Institutions.* All 1,135 two-year institutions, about two fifths of the nation's higher education institutions, are included in a single category.

5. *Professional Schools and Other Specialized Institutions.* The most heterogeneous group in the Carnegie Classification comprises the professional schools and other specialized institutions. These 576 institutions make up just under one fifth of the nation's higher education institutions. Included in this group are 51 medical schools and 29 other health professional schools that are located on a separate campus. No allied health schools are included, as none is located on a separate campus. Additional professional schools in this category include engineering, business, and teachers colleges.

References

Administration of Veterans Affairs. *May I Help You? Annual Report.* Washington, D.C.: Veterans Administration, 1977.

"AHA Survey Finds Hospitals Are Increasingly Turning to Shared Services as a Means of Holding Down Costs." *National Health Insurance Report,* 1978, *9*(5), 4.

American Council on Education. *A Fact Book on Higher Education, Third Issue, 1976.* Washington, D.C.: American Council on Education, 1976.

American Hospital Association. "Health Manpower Education and Training: Role and Responsibility of Hospitals and Other Health Care Agencies." *Statement,* 1974.

American Hospital Association. "Continuing Education for Personnel in Health Care Institutions." *Statement,* 1975.

American Hospital Association. "Mutual Responsibilities in Educating Health Manpower." *Guidelines,* 1976.

American Hospital Association. *Health Occupations Training Programs Administered by Hospitals, April 1976. A Directory.* Washington, D.C.: United States Government Printing Office, 1977a.

American Hospital Association. *Delivering Health Care in Rural America.* Chicago: American Hospital Association, 1977b.

American Hospital Association. *Hospital Statistics. 1978 Edition.* Chicago: American Hospital Association, 1978.

American Medical Association. *Allied Health Education Newsletter.* June 1978a, No. 110.

American Medical Association. "Medical Education in the United States: 78th Annual Report." *Journal of the American Medical Association,* 1978b, *240*(26, entire issue).

Anderson, P. W., Nunn, R. S., and Sedlacek, W. E. *Collegiate Programs in Allied Health Occupations.* Washington, D.C.: American Society of Allied Health Professions, 1976.

Anderson, P. W., and others. *Collegiate Programs in Allied Health Occupations, 1975-76.* Unpublished report. Washington, D.C.: American Society of Allied Health Professions, 1978.

Association Transfer Group. *College Transfer: Recommendations from Airlie House Conference: December 2-4, 1973.* Washington, D.C.: American Council on Education, 1974.

Bisconti, A. S., and Solmon, L. C. *College Education on the Job—The Graduates' Viewpoint.* Bethlehem, Pa.: CPC Foundation, 1976.

Bisconti, A. S., and Solmon, L. C. *Job Satisfaction After College—The Graduates' Viewpoint.* Bethlehem, Pa.: CPC Foundation, 1977.

Boatman, R. H., and Huther, J. W. (Eds.). *Allied Health Education. Transfer of Credit Recommendations of the North Carolina Articulation Project.* Chapel Hill, N.C.: University of North Carolina Press, 1974.

Borak, R., and Berdahl, R. *State Level Academic Program Review in Higher Education.* Denver, Colo.: Education Commission of the State, 1978.

Broski, D., and others. "Competency-Based Curriculum Development: A Pragmatic Approach." *Journal of Allied Health,* 1977, *6*(1), 38-44.

Bureau of the Census. *Estimates of the Population of the United States, by Age, Sex, and Race: 1970-1975.* Washington, D.C.: U.S. Government Printing Office, 1975.

Bureau of Health Manpower. *Education for the Allied Health Professions and Services: Report of the Allied Health Professions Education Subcommittee of the National Advisory Health Council.* Washington, D.C.: U.S. Government Printing Office, 1967.

Bureau of Health Manpower. *A Report to the President and Congress on the Status of Health Professions Personnel in the United States.* Advance Issue. Washington, D.C.: U.S. Government Printing Office, 1978.

Bureau of Labor Statistics. *Meeting Health Manpower Needs Through More Effective Use of Allied Health Workers.* Manpower Research Monograph No. 25. Washington, D.C.: U.S. Government Printing Office, 1973.

Bureau of Labor Statistics. *Occupational Outlook Handbook, 1978-79.* Washington, D.C.: U.S. Government Printing Office, 1978.

Burnett, C. N. "A Closer Look at Core." *Journal of Allied Health,* 1973, *2*(3), 107-112.

Carnegie Commission on Higher Education. *A Classification of Institutions of Higher Education.* Berkeley, Calif.: Carnegie Foundation for the Advancement of Teaching, 1973.

Center for Interdisciplinary Education in Allied Health. "Commission on Interprofessional Education and Practice." *Prospectus for Change,* 1979, *4*(3), 1-2.

Chronicle of Higher Education. "Earned Degrees Conferred, 1976." In *Chronicle of Higher Education Deskbook, 1978-79.* Washington, D.C.: Editorial Projects for Education, 1978a.

Chronicle of Higher Education. "Adult Continuing Education Programs: Noncredit Enrollment in 1975-76." In *Chronicle of Higher Education Deskbook, 1978-79.* Washington, D.C.: Editorial Projects for Education, 1978b.

Commission on Non-Traditional Study. *Diversity by Design.* San Francisco: Jossey-Bass, 1973.

Committee on Allied Health Education and Accreditation. *Allied Health Education Directory.* (7th ed.) Chicago: American Medical Association, 1978.

Connelly, T., Jr. "Interdisciplinary Education." Unpublished paper, National Commission on Allied Health Education, 1978.

Conners, M. A., Diener, T. J., Johnston, H. W., and Patterson, L. D. *Guide to Interinstitutional Arrangements: Voluntary and Statutory.* Washington, D.C.: American Association for Higher Education, 1974.

Council on Postsecondary Accreditation, American Council on Education, American Association of Collegiate Registrars and Admissions Officers. "Joint Statement on Transfer and Award of Credit." Mimeographed. Washington, D.C.: Council on Postsecondary Accreditation, 1978.

Davis, K., and Marshall, R. *Primary Health Care Services for Medically Underserved Populations.* Springfield, Va.: National Technical Information Service, 1977.

DuVal, M. K. "Allied Health Manpower from the Federal Viewpoint." *Journal of Allied Health,* 1972, *1*(1), 9-13.

Ellwood, P. M., McClure, W. J., and Rosala, J. C. *How Business Interacts with the Health Care System.* Washington, D.C.: National Chamber Foundation, 1978.

Erickson, E. W., and others. *Proprietary Business Schools and Community Colleges: Resource Allocation, Student Needs and Federal Policies.* Washington, D.C.: Inner City Fund, 1972.

Fuchs, V. R. "The Earnings of Allied Health Personnel—Are Health Workers Underpaid?" *Explorations in Economic Research,* 1976, *3*(3), 408-432.

Fuchs, V. R. "The Economics of Health in a Post-Industrial Society." *Public Interest,* 1979, *56,* 3-20.

Galambos, E. C. *Implications of Lengthened Health Education: Nursing and the Allied Health Fields.* Atlanta, Ga.: Southern Regional Education Board, 1979.

Goldstein, H. M., and Horowitz, M. A. *Health Personnel.* Germantown, Md.: Aspen Systems Corporation, 1977.

Hamburg, J. "Core Curriculum in Allied Health Education." *Journal of American Medical Association,* 1969, *210*(1), 111-113.

Harmon, W. W., and Quinones, M. A. "The Core Curriculum: A Response to the *Journal of Allied Health.*" *Journal of Allied Health,* 1974, *3*(1), 54-55.

Health Resources Administration. *The Supply of Health Manpower.* Washington, D.C.: U.S. Government Printing Office, 1974.

Holmstrom, E. I. *Trends and Career Changes of Students in the Health Fields: A Comparison with Other Disciplines.* Washington, D.C.: American Council on Education, 1973.

Holmstrom, E. I., and Bisconti, A. S. "Transfers From Junior to Senior Colleges. Final Report Submitted to the National Institute of Education." Mimeographed. Washington, D.C.: American Council on Education, 1974.

Holmstrom, E. I., Bisconti, A. S., and Kent, L. "National Commission Meets the Grass Roots: Concerns of Program Directors in Allied Health Education." *Journal of Allied Health,* 1978, *7*(4), 259-267.

Holmstrom, E. I., Knepper, P. R., and Kent, L. *Women and Minorities in Health Fields: A Trend Analysis of College Freshmen.* Vol. 1: *Freshmen Interested in the Health Professions.* Washington, D.C.: U.S. Government Printing Office, 1977a.

Holmstrom, E. I., Knepper, P. R., and Kent, L. *Women and Minorities in Health Fields: A Trend Analysis of College Freshmen.* Vol. 2: *Freshmen Interested in Nursing and Allied Health Fields.* Washington, D.C.: U.S. Government Printing Office, 1977b.

Holmstrom, E. I., Knepper, P. R., and Kent, L. *Women and Minorities in Health Fields: A Trend Analysis of College Freshmen.* Vol. 3: *A Comparison of Minority Aspirants to Health Careers.* Washington, D.C.: American Council on Education, 1977c.

Jacobsen, M. "Perceptions of Interdisciplinary Education Within Health Sciences Centers." Unpublished doctoral dissertation, Texas A & M University, 1977.

Jouette, M. L., and others. *Delineation of the Roles and Functions of Entry-Level Generalist Respiratory Therapy Practi-*

tioner. Dallas, Texas: American Association of Respiratory Therapy, 1978.

W. K. Kellogg Foundation. *Action Programs for Developing Allied Health Education.* Battle Creek, Mich.: W. K. Kellogg Foundation, 1977.

Kingston, R. D. "Graduate Level Experiences." In C. W. Ford (Ed.), *Clinical Education for the Allied Health Professions.* Saint Louis, Mo.: C. V. Mosby, 1978.

Kinsinger, R. E. "What This Country Doesn't Need is a Left Carotid Artery Technician or a Career-Based Response to the 'New Careers' Scramble." *Journal of Allied Health,* 1973, *2*(1), 10-15.

Kintzer, F. C. *Articulation and Transfer.* Los Angeles: ERIC Clearinghouse for Junior Colleges, UCLA, 1976.

Kirschner Associates. *A Descriptive Analysis of Health Programs Under CETA Legislation.* Phase I. Washington, D.C.: National Center for Health Services Research, 1977.

Kralovec, P., Williams, R., and Wilson, K. *1976 Survey of Health Occupations Training Programs in Hospitals.* Chicago: American Hospital Association, 1977.

Kriesberg, H. M., and others. *A Study of Dental Service Prepayment in the Private Sector.* Washington, D.C.: Robert R. Nathan Associates, 1978.

Lugenbeel, A. G. *Rural Allied Health Manpower Project 1974-1978. The Final Report.* Carbondale, Ill.: Southern Illinois University and the School of Technical Careers, 1979.

Marion, R. "Report on Health Science Education Outcome Survey." Mimeographed. Lexington, Ky.: Center for Interdisciplinary Education in Allied Health, 1978.

Martorana, S. V., and Nespoli, L. A. *Regionalism in American Postsecondary Education: Concepts and Practices.* University Park, Pa.: Center for the Study of Higher Education, Pennsylvania State University, 1978.

Mase, D. J. "Wither Now." Paper presented at the first annual meeting of the Association of Schools of Allied Health Professions, Miami Beach, Fla., November 1968.

Mase, D. J. "Foreword." In E. J. McTernan and R. O. Hawkins, Jr. (Eds.), *Educating Personnel for the Allied Health Professions and Services.* Saint Louis, Mo.: C. V. Mosby, 1972.

Mase, D. J. "National Health Planning and Resources Development Act of 1974. Public Law 93-641. Application to Allied Health Education." Unpublished paper, National Commission on Allied Health Education, 1968.

Moss, F. E., and Halamandaris, V. J. *Too Old, Too Sick, Too Bad: Nursing Homes in America.* Germantown, Md.: Aspen Systems Corporation, 1977.

National Center for Health Statistics. *Health–U.S. 1976-1977.* Washington, D.C.: U.S. Government Printing Office, 1977.

National Center for Health Statistics. *Health–U.S., 1978.* Washington, D.C.: U.S. Government Printing Office, 1978.

Newhouse, J. P., Phelps, C. E., and Schwarts, W. B. *Policy Options and the Impact of National Health Insurance.* Santa Monica, Calif.: Rand, 1974.

Ochsner, N. L., and Solmon, L. C. *College Education and Employment–The Recent Graduates.* Bethlehem, Pa.: CPC Foundation, 1979.

Office of Graduate Medical Education. *Interim Report of the Graduate Medical Education National Advisory Committee.* Washington, D.C.: U.S. Government Printing Office, 1979.

Ogden, H. G. "Section 1502 (10) Health Education and Public Law 93-641." In Health Resources Administration, *The Priorities of Section 1502.* Washington, D.C.: U.S. Government Printing Office, 1977.

Pellegrino, E. D. "Interdisciplinary Education in the Health Professions: Associations, Definitions, and Some Notes on Teams." In Institute of Medicine, *A Report of a Conference: Educating for the Health Team.* Washington, D.C.: National Academy of Sciences, 1972.

Pellegrino, E. D. "Allied Health Concept–Fact or Fiction?" *Journal of Allied Health,* 1974, *3*(2), 79-84.

Pellegrino, E. D. "The University of the Health Sciences." In Centre for Educational Research and Innovation, *Health, Higher Education, and the Community. Towards A Regional Health University.* Paris: Organization for Economic Cooperation and Development, 1977.

Pennell, M. Y., and Hoover, D. B. *Health Manpower Source Book 21.* Washington, D.C.: U.S. Government Printing Office, 1970.

Pennsylvania Department of Education. *Allied Health, Nursing, and Related Manpower Supply and Demand in Pennsylvania.* Harrisburg, Pa.: Pennsylvania Department of Education, 1977.

Perry, J. W. "Foreword." In C. W. Ford (Ed.), *Clinical Education for the Allied Health Professions.* Saint Louis, Mo.: C. V. Mosby, 1978.

Pruitt, J., and Ray, J. "Show Me the Way to Go Home." *Appalachia,* 1979, *12*(5), 55-56.

Public Health Service. *Forward Plan for Health: 1977-1981.* Washington, D.C.: U.S. Government Printing Office, 1975.

Public Health Service. *Credentialing Health Manpower.* Washington, D.C.: U.S. Government Printing Office, 1977.

Reinhardt, U. "Medicare: Its Financing and Future." *American Economic Review,* 1979, *69*(2), 279-283.

Richter, L., and Kosak, A. *Survey of Preparatory Education in Hospitals.* Chicago: American Hospital Association, 1975.

Roemer, M. I. *Health Care Systems in World Perspective.* Ann Arbor, Mich.: Health Administration Press, 1976.

Rosenfeld, M. H. "Organizing for Allied Health Education in Educational Institutions." In E. J. McTernan and R. O. Hawkins, Jr. (Eds.), *Educating Personnel for the Allied Health Professions and Services.* Saint Louis, Mo.: C. V. Mosby, 1972.

Rosinski, E. F. "An Approach to Developing a Competency-Based Curriculum—The California Story." In *Action Programs for Developing Allied Health Education.* Battle Creek, Mich.: W. K. Kellogg Foundation, 1977.

Scanlan, C. L. "Integrating Didactic and Clinical Education—High Patient Contact." In C. W. Ford (Ed.), *Clinical Education for the Allied Health Professions.* Saint Louis, Mo.: C. V. Mosby, 1978.

Smith, R. S. *The Occupational Safety and Health Act: Its Goals and Achievements.* Washington, D.C.: American Enterprise Institute for Public Policy Research, 1976.

Swift, J. L., Montalvo, R. A., and Ward, J. R. *HMOs. Their Potential Impact on Health Manpower Requirements.* Washington, D.C.: U.S. Government Printing Office, 1974.

Task Force on Allied Health Clinical Education. Vol. 1: *Final Report, National Assessment of Clinical Education of Allied Health Manpower.* Washington, D.C.: Booz-Allen and Hamilton, 1974.

Task Force on Proliferation. "Report on the Improvement of Nongovernmental Postsecondary Accreditation." Mimeographed. Washington, D.C.: Council on Postsecondary Accreditation, 1977.

Texas Coordinating Board. *Study of Nuclear Medicine Technology Education in Texas.* Austin: Texas Coordinating Board, 1978.

Tracka, M. R. "Hospitals Seek to Reduce Labor Costs." *Modern Health Care,* 1977, 7(8), 50.

U.S. Senate Committee on Human Resources. *Health Services and Primary Health Care Act of 1978, Report No. 95-860.* Washington, D.C.: U.S. Government Printing Office, 1978.

Weiss, J. H. "The Changing Job Structure of Health Manpower." Unpublished doctoral dissertation, Harvard University, 1966.

Wilms, W. W. "The Effectiveness of Public and Proprietary Occupational Training." Mimeographed. Berkeley, Calif.: Center for Research and Development in Higher Education, 1974.

Wynder, E. L., and Kristein, M. M. "Suppose We Died Young, Late in Life." *Journal of the American Medical Association,* 1977, *238*(14), 1507.

Youn, T. I., and Thompson, R. S. "A Summary and Analysis of the National Commission's Survey of Noncollegiate Institutions." Mimeographed. Washington, D.C.: National Commission on the Financing of Postsecondary Education, 1974.

Index

D

E

Q

R